JUVENILE ASTHMA

Comforting communication from a parent, especially when a child is upset, angry, or fearful—emotions that go hand in hand with asthma attacks—is the gift of **reflexology**. And **thumb-walking** helps break up congestion and relax bronchial muscles.

NONORGANIC ALLERGIES

Chemicals, pesticides, and air pollution trigger headaches, eczema, coughing, and itchy eyes. **Herbal teas** or **herbal-based emollients and oils** combat a sick environment and build up your resistance to chronic industrial pollutants.

HAY FEVER

Every year millions buy over-the-counter remedies or head for desensitization injections. **Homeopathic** medicine focuses on curing the underlying immune system imbalance and can bring relief to sneezing, congested victims.

SKIN ALLERGIES

Emotions and stress are major factors in baffling, often seemingly incurable skin allergies. **Meditation** can make you less susceptible to allergens . . . in a recommended routine that takes just a few minutes a day.

PLUS

**ALLERGIC RHINITIS · JUVENILE ALLERGIES
ADULT ASTHMA · FOOD ALLERGIES
ALLERGIES AND ADDICTION**

THE DELL NATURAL MEDICINE LIBRARY
Health and Healing the Natural Way

LOOK FOR THESE OTHER TITLES IN
THE DELL NATURAL MEDICINE LIBRARY:

Stress, Anxiety, and Depression
Women's Health
Chronic Pain

THE NATURAL WAY
OF HEALING

ASTHMA AND ALLERGIES

The Natural Medicine Collective

Dr. Brian Fradet, D.C.
(Coordinating Panelist, Chiropractic)
Dr. William Bergman, M.D. *(Homeopathy)*
Brian Clement *(Nutrition)*
Elaine Retholtz, L.Ac. *(Acupuncture)*
Dr. James Lawrence Thomas, Ph.D. *(Psychology)*
Dr. Maurice H. Werness, Jr., N.D. *(Naturopathy)*

with
Gary McLain

A DELL BOOK

PRODUCED BY THE PHILIP LIEF GROUP, INC.

Published by
Dell Publishing
a division of
Bantam Doubleday Dell Publishing Group, Inc.
1540 Broadway
New York, New York 10036

Note to the Reader:

This book is not for the purpose of self-diagnosis or self-treatment, and should be used only in conjunction with the advice of your personal doctor. Readers should consult an appropriate medical professional in all matters relating to their health.

Produced by The Philip Lief Group, Inc., 9 West 20th Street, New York, New York

Copyright © 1995 by The Philip Lief Group, Inc.

ISBN: 0-440-21662-1

Printed in the United States of America

Published simultaneously in Canada

April 1995

10 9 8 7 6 5 4 3 2 1

RAD

Contents

Introduction 1

CHAPTER ONE • *What Is Natural Medicine?* 7

CHAPTER TWO • *Natural Therapies: An Overview* 20

CHAPTER THREE • *A First Look at Asthma and Allergy* 68

CHAPTER FOUR • *Allergic Rhinitis and Hay Fever* 128

CHAPTER FIVE • *Juvenile Allergies* 174

CHAPTER SIX • *Adult Asthma* 208

CHAPTER SEVEN • *Juvenile Asthma* 246

CHAPTER EIGHT • *Inorganic Allergies and Chronic Industrial Irritants* 273

CHAPTER NINE • *Skin Allergies and Eczema* 308

CHAPTER TEN • *Food Allergies* 335

Glossary 376

Natural Medicine Resources 378

Herb Sources 382

Acupressure Points 384

The Natural Medicine Collective: Biographies 388

Index 391

Introduction

Asthma and Allergies, part of The Natural Way of Healing Series, is aimed at expanding your options for treating your asthma and allergy symptoms through a range of natural medicine alternatives, some relatively new, and some based on traditions that have been in existence for centuries.

Literally millions and millions of people suffer from some form of allergy or asthma, resulting in symptoms that range from a stomachache to skin rash to violent sneezing, coughing, and wheezing. Both asthma and allergies are complex in that they are often difficult to predict as well as control.

No two individuals have the same experience. Allergy symptoms can appear occasionally, seasonably, or in some cases, be an everyday occurrence. Sometimes the cause is mysterious, with the symptoms seeming to appear out of nowhere. Other times they are more predictable, such as when a cat walks into the room and those with dander allergies immediately begin sneezing and coughing. To further complicate the picture, the severity of an allergic reaction can range from mildly annoying to life threatening.

Allergies may or may not be related to asthma. Individuals who have asthma, like allergy sufferers, often experience symptoms that seem like surprise attacks, sometimes triggered by factors such as stress or major changes in the weather. And also like allergies, asthma symptoms can quickly progress from mild to severe.

The medical establishment has made great strides in developing treatments and emergency procedures, allowing many with severe asthma and allergies to lead active lives. Yet treating asthma and allergies is, to a great extent, an inexact science. Many continue to suffer from occasional symptoms that can greatly interfere with day-to-day activities.

As a result, a multimillion-dollar over-the-counter drug industry has emerged to offer creams, nasal sprays, and pills that provide some level of symptom relief. Over-the-counter medication can be helpful in the short term, through reducing some of the more obvious symptoms. Sooner or later, however, the symptoms reappear. Furthermore, many experts fear that medications based on chemicals may interfere with the body's natural ability to fight off disease. Nasal sprays, for example, can interfere with the normal functioning of the sinuses and even become addictive. As a result, the treatment may in fact contribute to the problem. Or the treatment may not help at all.

Increasingly, natural medicine is being explored by those suffering from asthma and allergy. This interest is in part the result of a growing awareness of the role of factors other than heredity in the development of these conditions. Natural medicine is based on a holistic view of asthma and allergy. For example, a diet filled with food additives, constant exposure to air pollution, and living in stressful, noisy environments are factors that are also believed to be contributors to asthma and allergy. Thus, rather than simply providing temporary symptom relief, natural medicine seeks to treat the whole person, physically, emotionally, and even spiritually.

Asthma and Allergies provides information on a range of natural medicine options, ranging from ancient Chinese medical practices such as acupuncture and acupressure, to botanical medicine, aromatherapy, and homeopathy. The book also includes practices such as massage and reflexology, as well as meditation and visualization. Botanical remedies, for example, can provide relief of symptoms such as wheezing or itchy skin. These remedies can also help bring the various systems of the body back into balance, which helps to prevent the occurrence of symptoms in the future. Meditation, visualization, and other alternatives can be helpful in reducing the tension that often precedes asthma and allergy symptoms.

Asthma and Allergies is arranged by different types of asthma and allergies, including adult and juvenile asthma, food allergy, and skin allergy. Within each chapter is a brief discussion of how the condition develops and what the symptoms look like. Alternative natural medicine treatments, within each chapter, are arranged alphabetically. Each of these natural medicine alternatives is described in terms of how it works in treating your asthma and allergy condition, what you can expect from working with a practitioner of this form of natural medicine, and wherever possible, remedies and techniques you can try at home. These natural medicine alternatives were written under the guidance of The Natural Medicine Collective, each member an expert in one specific natural medicine approach.

Read Chapters 1 and 2 first, to gain a better understanding of natural medicine and the broad range of approaches available to you. Chapter 3 will provide you with a foundation for applying natural medicine in treating your asthma and allergy symptoms. The immune system is discussed, which is where allergy conditions have their roots; the major natural medicine approaches, and their applications, are described in depth. You may want to read all of the chapters that follow, or only the ones that focus on your specific condition.

Natural medicine can be helpful both in preventing and treating minor asthma and allergy symptoms, but can also complement whatever treatment you are receiving from your physician. In fact, many physicians are increasingly open to, and even recommend, natural medicine treatments as an adjunct to conventional medical treatment. Allergy desensitization injections might be accompanied by meditation, for example, to aid in reducing stress. Homeopathic remedies, or acupuncture, might be prescribed in addition to a plan for treating symptoms that have become severe. Additionally, members of the medical establishment are placing increasing emphasis on proper diet and exercise in treating illness, as well as recognizing the importance of a positive outlook.

Natural medicine is a complementary form of treatment. Some approaches, like natural medicine and meditation, work together, while others may not be natural complements. In any case, your initial point of reference is your physician.

FIRST: A CAUTION

Asthma and allergy can be life threatening. For example, an allergic reaction can progress to anaphylactic shock, with symptoms that include headache, itchy skin, vomiting, nausea, sneezing and coughing, abdominal cramps, shortness of breath, convulsions, and loss of consciousness, as well as other symptoms. These symptoms, if untreated, can lead to death. Furthermore, asthma can progress to loss of consciousness and death.

Because of the potential dangers associated with

asthma and allergy, it is important to be under the care of a medical doctor. A physician can help you to assess your own potential for life-threatening symptoms, and provide you with both medication and guidance on what to do in case of an emergency. Consider natural medicine alternatives for their potential in helping you reduce both the severity of your symptoms as well as the frequency with which symptoms occur. Don't make any decisions about alternative medicine without first consulting your physician.

CHAPTER ONE

What Is Natural Medicine?

Acid rain . . . the disappearing ozone layer . . . smog . . . radiation . . . contaminated well water . . . It has become evident, from media reports as well as from personal experiences, that our increasing knowledge and technology can both help to advance society as well as wreak havoc on our lives. In a similar way, as the science of medicine has become more technical and has made great strides in treating many illnesses, it also has become more and more manipulative of and invasive to the human body. Unnecessary surgeries, excessive medication, life-support mechanisms . . . all of these alter the natural processes of health and illness, life and death. One cannot deny the value of surgery and medication in treating certain ailments and diseases, but it seems that we often lose sight of the body's power and ability, with the proper care and nurturing, to heal itself.

This notion of healing oneself is at the root of natural medicine philosophy. As more people witness the harmful effects of technology and the overuse of conventional modern medicine, they are turning to alternatives that are less invasive and disruptive of the body's natural processes. The new "health-consciousness craze" of the 1990s is all around us. People are striving to eat the right foods and maintain their proper weight; more people have made exercise a regular part of their daily routine; and some have discovered the benefits of relaxation and meditation, two elements that are particularly vital in our fast-paced, hectic lives.

You might grant that diet, exercise, and stress reduction are all well and good, yet doubt that they are a sufficient means of curing specific illnesses. How can riding the Lifecycle for twenty minutes three times a week possibly help chronic acid indigestion? The missing link is the mind: Proper care of your body helps create a healthy mind, and a balanced mind leads to a healthy body. They are interrelated; some believe they are one and the same. As a society, we are skeptical—we like to have things proven through testing and experimentation, and we like to see the facts. The brain and neurological system can be viewed as the physical embodiment of the mind, and this is true to the extent that scientists and doctors can measure and test these vital organs. The mind, however, is more than a mass of nerves, hormones, and electrical impulses. It represents an invisible, intangible, yet extremely powerful energy that, unfortunately, we often are too quick to dismiss.

Throughout history the mind has been viewed as something that must be mastered and controlled, otherwise one might "lose one's mind" or "go out of one's mind." An inability to control one's mind signified personal weakness to many people. It is useful, however, to think of the mind not as something to be controlled lest one go mad, but as energy to be harnessed and used to restore and maintain overall health. Indeed, this is the underlying philosophy of the practice of natural medicine.

Vis medicatrix naturae—the healing power of nature— this is the premise of natural medicine, which involves the use of an array of noninvasive, natural therapies to help restore balance to the body and thus help the system to heal itself. These therapies, which will be discussed individually in Chapter 2, include Oriental medicine, homeopathy, hydrotherapy, botanical medicine, physical medicine, psychotherapy, biofeedback, and nutrition. Natural medicine discourages the use of treatments that weaken the body's innate ability to heal itself, and although a person sometimes requires more than natural remedies, the natural medicine practitioner will always try to use the least invasive treatment possible.

Natural medicine functions from a holistic point of view; that is, your whole being is treated, rather than simply the part of your body that is sick. Natural medicine practitioners will take into consideration not only your obvious and immediate symptoms but lifestyle, psychological factors, and other physical imbalances that may be present. They believe that illness affects the whole person—physically, emotionally, and mentally—and that imbalances within and among these three spheres will cause a person to exhibit symptoms of sickness. Natural medicine requires you to become involved in your own healing and to claim responsibility for your own health. Doctors have long been considered teachers of a certain kind, and natural medicine practitioners continue the tradition of educating their patients to become more aware of their own bodies, emotions, and minds and to help the self-healing process along.

Natural medicine strives for a balance between mind and body. If appropriate and necessary, various therapies can be used concurrently, or they can be used to supplement standard medical treatment if the case warrants it. The fact is that no one remedy or therapy—whether it is conventional or alternative—can work for everyone all of the time. The key is to explore your options and use the treatment that is most successful in treating your overall health and well-being.

Natural therapies are gaining popularity as people increasingly realize that conventional medicine cannot always offer all the answers or cures. According to a study published in the *New England Journal of Medicine* in January 1993, approximately one-third of all Americans used alternative medicine therapies in 1990, including relaxation techniques, massage, macrobiotic diets, spiritual healing, self-help groups, biofeedback, acupuncture, hypnosis, chiropractic, herbal medicine, and homeopathy. Patients spent $10.3 billion on alternative health care in 1990, and 90 percent of the treatments were sought by patients without the advice or suggestion of their regular physician.

The mainstream health-care industry, likewise, is changing to keep up with the growing demand for alternative medicine. The National Institutes of Health, at the urging of Congress, established an Office for the Study of Unconventional Medicine Practices and an Office of Alternative Medicine in 1992. Some conventional physicians have incorporated natural medicine philosophy and technique into their own practices. Insurance companies such as the American Western Life Insurance Company of California, the Mutual of Omaha Insurance Company, Blue Cross of Washington and Alaska, and the New Jersey–based Prudential have extended coverage to include natural therapies. Clearly, natural medicine is becoming more popular as patients seek alternative treatments to those offered in Western medicine.

DIFFERENCES BETWEEN
CONVENTIONAL AND ALTERNATIVE
MEDICINE

Standard, conventional, or orthodox medicine, also called *allopathy*, defines health as the absence of disease. This definition is based on a negative. In contrast, holistic medicine concurs with the definition of health used by the World Health Organization (WHO), which posits that it is a state of complete physical, mental, and social well-being.

The allopathic and holistic definitions of health differ greatly in regard to the diagnosis and treatment of illness. People who use conventional medicine usually do not seek treatment until they become ill; there is little emphasis on preventive treatment. Holistic medicine, in contrast, focuses on preventing illness and maintaining health. The best illustration of this approach is the fact that ancient Chinese doctors were paid only when their patients were healthy, not if they became ill.

Natural medicine, which follows a holistic approach, views illness and disease as an imbalance of the mind and body that is expressed on the physical, emotional, and mental levels of a person. Although allopathy does recognize that many physical symptoms have mental components (for example, emotional stress might promote an ulcer or chronic headaches), its approach is generally to suppress the symptoms, both physical and psychological. Natural medicine assesses the symptoms as a sign or reflection of a deeper instability within the person, and it tries to restore the physical and mental harmony that will then alleviate the symptoms.

Except for cases of severe physical trauma, most illness derives from a level of susceptibility that varies in different people. For instance, some people seem to catch every cold and flu virus that goes around, while others can go for years without so much as a sniffle or a cough. The level of susceptibility reflects the deepest state of one's being. Bacteria and germs, as well as carcinogens, allergens, and other toxins, are agents of illness waiting to prey on a susceptible host. These stimuli alone do not cause illness, but rather induce specific symptoms in susceptible persons. Certain bacteria are known to be associated with certain diseases, and there are bacteria living within our bodies all of the time. Hence, if bacteria were the cause of illness, we would probably be sick all of the time. Instead, illness occurs when an imbalance in the body allows the bacteria to reproduce uncontrollably. Natural medicine usually views this uncontrolled growth as a manifestation of disease, not a cause of it. Natural medicine practitioners believe that preventive medicine, or therapies designed to maintain and enhance health, can reduce people's susceptibility and therefore the frequency with which they become ill.

Because of the fundamental differences in the way that allopathic and alternative physicians define and view health and illness, they also assess and treat their patients in very different ways. Alternative practitioners believe that people can use the power and positive energy of their minds to defend themselves against disease. Symptoms, therefore, are not caused by illness, but reflect the body's best attempt to heal itself. Since allopathic doctors believe that symptoms are caused by disease, they also believe that alleviating the symptoms will foster cure. In contrast, the natural medicine practitioner will claim that suppressing symptoms fails to address the underlying cause of illness and, in fact, can drive the illness deeper into the body, causing more profound symptoms to develop.

For example, if a child has a fever, an allopathic doctor might prescribe acetaminophen. Although this can help to bring the fever down, it is not curing the illness, which must run its course. An alternative practitioner, on the other hand, would consider the fever to be an indication that the body is fighting the illness. A high temperature makes the body unsuitable for bacteria to grow, and so it is the body's natural defense against the infection. Of course, an excessively high fever can be dangerous and should be treated so as to reduce it.

The difference between allopathic and natural treatments also can be seen in relation to the common cold. An allopathic doctor might suggest using an antihistamine to dry up a runny nose. However, natural medicine believes that the flow of mucus, and indeed all bodily secretions, is significant to the healing process, as it rids the body of toxic substances. If you are the kind of person who likes the quick remedy—that magic syrup or pill—and does not want to endure the discomforts of illness in the recovery process, you will have to assess whether natural medicine is appropriate for you. All of the alternative therapies discussed in this book require that your mind be open to their philosophies and that you become an active participant in your own recovery and health promotion.

In allopathy, diagnostic testing is vital in order for the doctor to name and categorize the disease and to treat it. Often these tests are done routinely, sometimes for the purpose of protecting the doctor rather than actually to help the patient. Some diagnostic tests, such as excessive X rays, or the use of powerful drugs can even cause sickness, referred to as iatrogenic illness, meaning "doctor-caused."

Although modern holistic doctors might use some standard diagnostic tests, they are more concerned with the individual's life circumstances. When you visit an alternative practitioner for the first time, he or she will consult at length with you, or "take the case," as it is called. During this initial visit, which can last more than an hour, the doctor will interview you, making notes about your verbal and nonverbal communication. The practitioner will be careful not to compare you with another patient, as each individual is unique. The doctor will record his or her observations of you as well as your complaints and concerns and will most likely ask questions to better individualize the case. If you are seeking help for an acute illness, the doctor probably will focus on symptoms and feelings that have changed since you became ill. If you are complaining of a chronic ailment, the doctor will want to know as much as possible about your life and history. Conventional diagnostic testing can be useful in certain cases, but the alternative doctor's practice of "taking the case" allows him or her to get at the deeper source of your problem, rather than just treating your symptoms.

Natural medicine operates on Hippocrates' theory of *primum non nocere*, or "first do no harm." The goal is to treat illness with noninvasive, harmless remedies that invoke the body's innate healing powers. Natural medicine involves a comprehensive view of health, illness, treatment, and cure that meets the need of each individual person and helps to restore and maintain balance of the body and mind.

In some cases, natural treatment can suffice to cure an illness, but other times allopathic treatments are required. If this is the case, alternative treatments can still be used to enhance the effectiveness of allopathic medicine, providing maximum healing for the individual. Healthy individuals also can pursue natural medicine regimens to maintain and enhance their physical, emotional, and mental well-being.

HISTORY OF NATURAL
MEDICINE IN THE WEST

The word *naturopathy* was not used until the late nineteenth century, although its philosophy originated with Hippocrates, whose school of medicine existed around 400 B.C. Earlier people believed that disease was caused by supernatural powers. Hippocrates devised the theory that everything natural had a rational basis and that the causes of disease could be found in natural elements, such as air, water, or food. He also believed in *vis medicatrix naturae*, or the healing power of nature, and that the body had its own ability to heal itself.

The years from 1780 to 1850 marked the Age of Heroic Medicine. During this time, "heroic" treatments, such as bleeding, intestinal purgings, and blistering of the skin, were used to cure patients of their ills. These treatments were painful and harmful, and they often made patients worse, or even induced death. It was believed that bleeding, accomplished by lancing a vein or using leeches, removed impurities from the body. Intestinal purgings were performed by using mercuric chloride, which today we know causes severe metal poisoning; vomiting was induced by using other poisonous substances. The Age of Heroic Medicine was male-dominated and elitist, excluding women and nonconventional doctors. Some physicians who opposed heroic medicine practiced alternatives such as herbalism.

In 1810, a German doctor named Samuel Hahnemann (1755–1843) became disenchanted with the standard medicine of his day and began the practice of homeopathy. *Homeopathy* is derived from two Greek roots meaning "similar" and "disease, suffering." It is a philosophy of health and cure that is based on the principle that like cures like. That is, natural substances that produce particular symptoms in a healthy person can cure a sick person with those same symptoms.

Hahnemann did not actually originate the philosophy that like cures like; Hippocrates and others also had explored this concept previously. However, he did develop the theory into a viable alternative medical practice, homeopathy, which is discussed in greater detail in Chapter 2.

When Hahnemann died at the age of eighty-eight in 1843, he had many followers in Europe. The first homeopathic doctor came to the United States in 1828. In 1836, the Hahnemann Medical College opened in Philadelphia, and the first national medical society, the American Institute of Homeopathy, was established in 1844. As people began to react against heroic medical practices and politics, the Popular Health Movement was formed. It called for the repeal of all medical licensing laws, which was achieved by the end of the 1840s. This allowed physicians to practice whatever form of medicine they believed in. It was in this atmosphere that homeopathy flourished in the United States and set the stage for other alternative medicines, such as naturopathy, to take root.

Realizing that they were losing their foothold, the allopaths organized the American Medical Association (AMA) in 1846. While attacking homeopathy, they tried to give allopathy a more positive definition by claiming the word was based on German roots meaning "all therapies." Allopathy thus began to allow that a variety of remedies could be effective in treating a disease. The AMA required state medical societies to expel homeopaths and alternative healers, and in the 1860s, charges often were brought against allopaths who associated with these doctors. Allopaths began to wrest control of city hospitals and boards of health, and they succeeded in reestablishing licensing laws in all states. As the Popular Health Movement dissolved, alternative healers virtually were driven out of practice and denied any political influence.

By the 1880s, the homeopathic movement was being destroyed not only by the AMA but by its own internal philosophical divisions. Two groups of homeopaths emerged: those who were pure homeopaths, called Hahnemannians, and a larger, more modern group that included allopathic practices in their work and that wanted to work with allopathic doctors rather than against them.

Dr. John Scheel of New York City coined the word *naturopathy* in 1895 to connote "nature cure." The earliest forms of natural treatments and preventions included good hygiene and hydrotherapy. Naturopathy began to be pursued in full force in the United States in 1902 by Benedict Lust, who had emigrated from Germany in 1892. He had grown dissatisfied with conventional medicine and was intrigued by the European health spas, especially their treatment involving water cures and fasts. By the end of the nineteenth century, water cure was recognized as a vital healing therapy and referred to by the term *hydrotherapy*.

Lust intended to practice and teach hydrotherapy in the United States. Soon, however, his followers broadened their practices and healing philosophy to include an array of modalities, such as nutritional therapy, herbal medicine, homeopathy, spinal manipulation, exercise, hydrotherapy, electrotherapy, and stress management. Lust believed that in order to achieve good health, people should eliminate excessive consumption of toxic substances (such as caffeine, drugs, and alcohol), exercise, strive for a good mental attitude, and amend their lifestyles to include natural remedies such as fasting, proper diet, hydrotherapy, mud baths, chiropractic, and the like. He opened the American School of Naturopathy in New York City, which graduated its first class in 1902.

Natural medicine became very popular in the United States in the early twentieth century until the mid-1930s. At that point, conventional medicine again began to rise to prominence and popularity because of several factors. First, chemical and drug industries, which benefit more economically from allopathic than natural medicine, financially supported foundations that subsidized conventional medical schools. Second, orthodox medicine began to use less harmful treatments, and advances in health-care technology, particularly in surgery, convinced the public that conventional medicine was superior to natural medicine. The orthodox medical arena again began passing legislation that either limited or prohibited alternative health-care systems from flourishing.

Within the past two decades, since the 1970s, natural medicine has begun to take hold again. Realizing that allopathic medicine may not have all of the answers or cures for their ills, people are seeking alternative treatments. As people begin to recognize the devastating contaminating effects of some technology on air, water, and food, they are also beginning to take action against such harmful practices. Finally, as the connection between the mind and body becomes ever more apparent, people are willing to make major lifestyle changes in order to protect and maintain their sense of physical and emotional balance. This is what natural medicine is all about and it is why more and more people are realizing the long-term benefits of alternative medical treatments.

LOCATING A NATURAL MEDICINE PRACTITIONER

One of the best ways to find a good alternative practitioner is to be referred by one of his or her patients, though you might not be fortunate enough to find one in this way. At the end of this book is a list of Natural Medicine Resources. Contact the listed organizations. Often they can make referrals to practitioners in your area, or they may have membership directories available.

When consulting a practitioner, interview him or her to learn as much as you can about the person and his or her practice. As a result of the interview, you will feel more comfortable seeking help from this person if you decide to do so, and that level of trust and comfort will facilitate a beneficial outcome for your treatment. The American Holistic Medical Association can send you a publication, *How to Choose a Holistic Health Practitioner*. The organization's address is listed in the Natural Medicine Resources section. Following are some questions to ask a practitioner you interview:

- What schools did you attend and what is the extent of your training?
- What licenses or certificates do you hold?
- How long have you been in practice?
- What are your diagnostic and treatment procedures?
- What are the fees involved? What is the length of treatment or number of sessions proposed?
- Have you written any articles or books? (If so, they may be worth reading.)

CHAPTER TWO

Natural Therapies:
An Overview

ORIENTAL MEDICINE

Oriental medicine defines health not as an absence of disease, as in Western medicine, but as a total state of well-being. It requires that the body be free from physical pain, but also encompasses the totality of the individual's thoughts, emotions, and beliefs. Health, in Eastern philosophy, is a state of mind and a way of life. Illness results from going against the natural laws of Heaven and Earth.

Oriental medicine began at least three thousand years ago, and has developed progressively as a science since approximately A.D. 200. It continues to flourish in the Eastern countries today, and many aspects of Oriental medicine are beginning to gain popularity as alternative treatments in the West. Oriental medicine involves several healing therapies, including acupuncture, herbs, nutrition, exercise (such as tai chi chuan and other martial arts), massage, and manipulation.

Taoism, Confucianism, and Buddhism are the underlying philosophies of Chinese medicine. According to Taoism, health reflects a harmony in Heaven, which is achieved through the balance of external and internal forces. A unity exists within the diversity of nature—a universal energy that exists in all things. This energy, called *chi,* is very difficult to describe. It has been explained as matter on the verge of becoming energy, while at the same time it is also energy on the verge of becoming matter. Everything in the universe is a result of the never-ending condensation of *chi* into matter and dispersion of *chi* into energy. In terms of Chinese medicine, *chi* needs to be understood in two ways. First, it nourishes the mind and body and has been described as the life force. Second, *chi* is produced by and indicates the function of the various *zang/fu,* or "spheres of function." *Zang/fu* refers not to a specific organ, such as the liver, but to the totality of body functions associated with the liver. Stomach *chi,* therefore, refers to various stomach functions, such as the transportation of food essences. The Chinese believe that *chi* flows throughout the human body. Health reflects a free flow of *chi,* but if the energy is imbalanced—if there is a blockage, an excess, or a deficiency of *chi* in specific body parts or organs—disease and illness occur.

Taoism also recognizes two opposite yet complementary qualities to all aspects of physical being. The philosophy derives from the notion that the universe was originally a ball of *chi* surrounded by chaos. When this mass of energy finally settled, it divided into the two opposing yet complementary qualities called *yin* and *yang.* Yin represents qualities that are negative, contractive, dark, small, of the right side, interior, of the nature of Earth. Yang, in contrast, is positive, expansive, light, big, of the left side, surface, of the nature of Heaven. All objects, animals, peoples, times, and places are a combination of yin and yang. It is believed that people are born with perfect yin and yang balance that is later thrown off kilter. Chinese doctors designate certain organs as being either of yin or yang qualities, and so are the foods and medicinal herbs that would be used to treat ailments of these organs.

Practitioners of Chinese medicine and philosophers believe in a dynamic cycle of evolution known as the five-element theory. All things are classified according to the five elements of wood, fire, earth, metal, and water. The body's organs are also characterized by the five elements; for example, the spleen and stomach are of the earth, and the lung and large intestine are of metal. These five elements are in a state of constant change and interact with one another. Doctors believe that organs affect other organs according to the elements. For instance, wood generates fire; therefore, the activity of the liver, which is characterized by wood, generates the activity of the heart, which is a fire organ. The relationships between the elements show doctors the direction in which *chi* flows within the body.

Just as the Chinese views about health differ from Western notions, so do their ideas about human anatomy. Chinese doctors identify twelve organs, or the *zang/fu*, which do not correspond directly to organs as we know them. Remember that *zang/fu* refers not to a specific organ, but to all of the body functions associated with that organ. This way of looking at the body probably evolved because ancient Chinese tradition prohibited the opening of corpses. Therefore, rather than developing a more detailed, concrete knowledge of anatomy, scientists and doctors focused on body functions instead of specific organs. The result is a more holistic understanding of function that embraces physical, mental, and emotional aspects.

Chinese medicine requires that the flow of *chi* in the body be influenced or moved, either by the practitioner or by the patient, so as to restore its balance. The flow of *chi* can be impeded by poor nutrition; lack of exercise; mental stress; fatigue; bad posture and breathing; pollution; physical growths such as tumors; or trauma, including those that result in scar tissue. A deficiency in *chi* can cause fatigue, depression, and various physical ailments. Excess *chi* might be responsible for hypertension, migraine headaches, or some types of arthritis. If the natural flow of *chi* through the body is altered in any way, a host of ailments could occur.

Chi flows through the body in fourteen pathways called meridians. The geography of the human body, as viewed by Eastern doctors, is based on these pathways as well as the *zang/fu* (organs) and bowels, and is very different from Western concepts of anatomy and physiology. Twelve of the meridians pass through a major organ and are linked to other meridians, so that all body parts have access to *chi*.

Practitioners of Oriental medicine examine and diagnose their patients in a way that is quite different from the quick, routine examinations and consultations patients in the West are accustomed to. There is careful questioning and observation of the patient, as well as monitoring of the patient's pulse. This is not pulse-checking as we know it, however. Rather, it is a fine art of detecting several layers of pulses in order to determine which body spheres are suffering. The doctor will take a pulse using the first three fingers of his or her hand, checking the patient's wrists with both light and firm pressure. The doctor will also identify pulses under each finger at both pressure levels—a total of six pulses for each wrist. Each pulse correlates with a specific body function sphere.

Acupuncture

One of the major Oriental healing arts is acupuncture, which involves the insertion of needles at specific points on the body. These special points are located along the various meridians, twelve of which correspond to a particular organ. It is indeed an art as well as a science to be able to locate the precise point at which a needle should be inserted. If it is not placed in the right position, the procedure will not have the desired effect. The purpose of acupuncture is to move or restore the flow of *chi* through the insertion of the needles along the meridians relevant to the illness.

The needles are inserted quickly and left in place for several minutes. Sometimes the doctor will just pierce the skin, while other times the needle will be inserted up to an inch deep. The doctor might twirl the needle to increase stimulation. Another process of stimulating the acupuncture points is called *moxabustion*. In one method of moxabustion, the needles' heads are wrapped with dry *moxa* (Chinese wormwood) and burned. The needle conducts the heat into the acupuncture point. In yet another process, called electroacupuncture, the doctor connects each needle to a small machine that stimulates the needles with a low electrical pulse.

To those people raised with Western medical treatments, acupuncture is often viewed as a superstitious practice. The thought of having needles inserted into various regions of the body, even places as delicate as the face, can make even the staunchest Westerner squeamish. Those who have experienced acupuncture, however, claim that it is a painless, effective treatment for many illnesses. An acupuncture patient probably will feel a slight sensation when the needles are inserted. As the acupuncture works, the patient also might feel the presence of *chi* at the sites of the needles or the movement of *chi* in the body.

All this discussion about *chi* and influencing its movement through the body may be difficult for you to accept. Western scientists and doctors have devised several theories to explain why acupuncture works, especially when it is used to alleviate pain. One theory is based on the fact that the body produces endorphins and enkephalins, natural painkilling chemicals that can also help allergies and depression and can facilitate healing. Stimulating acupuncture points increases the body's production of endorphins and enkephalins. Another theory to explain acupuncture is that it has a placebo effect if the patient truly believes that it will help. Still another is based on the fact that some scientists and doctors feel that our vital energy is not *chi*, as the Chinese know it, but rather electricity. Acupuncture affects the way electricity travels along the meridians. Kirlian photography, which illustrates bioelectricity, provides evidence that this is a viable theory. The picture of a hand before and after acupuncture reveals an increased flow of electricity after the treatment. Finally, the gate theory of pain also is used to explain acupuncture. According to this theory, the body contains neuropathway "gates" along the spinal cord leading to the brain. Acupuncture closes the gates so that messages of pain do not reach the brain.

From a Chinese medicine point of view, acupuncture works as a result of regulating the flow of *chi* and blood. There is a Chinese expression, "There is no pain if there is free flow; if there is pain, there is no free flow."

Acupuncture has been shown to be an effective analgesic and has even been used instead of anesthetics during surgery. The stimulation of the acupuncture points in order to produce an analgesic effect causes the brain to release endorphins, which are the body's natural painkilling chemicals. Although Chinese doctors might use anesthetics during an operation, using acupuncture as an analgesic necessitates using only a fraction of the dose that a surgical patient in the West would receive. This is especially important for people who are sensitive to painkillers and anesthesia, as acupuncture is a harmless, safe way to treat pain.

Acupuncture can be an effective treatment for both terminal and nonterminal illnesses. A therapy that can be used alone or in combination with another treatment, it is also useful in dealing with the side effects of conventional medicine.

If you are considering acupuncture as a healing therapy, try to get a referral from an acupuncture society or school, from the pain clinic at your local hospital, or from someone who has experienced the treatment firsthand. Investigate the training and experience of the doctor until you are satisfied with his or her qualifications. Licensing varies by state: Some license independent practitioners, while others restrict practice to medical doctors (those with an M.D. degree) or allow acupuncturists to work only under such a doctor's supervision. Contact the American Association of Acupuncture and Oriental Medicine, the National Commission for the Certification of Acupuncturists, or the National Accreditation Commission for Schools and Colleges of Acupuncture and Oriental Medicine (see the Natural Medicine Resources section) for information regarding licensing requirements in your state and for more information about acupuncture.

Visits to an acupuncturist range in cost from $35 to $75. Some insurance companies do cover the cost of acupuncture, but many still do not, and some will cover only those treatments recommended by a conventional doctor. Be sure to check your policy regarding your coverage for acupuncture.

When you visit an acupuncturist, make sure that the doctor uses either presterilized disposable needles or an autoclave, which is a sterilizing machine. An autoclave is the only effective way to sterilize needles and other medical or dental instruments sufficiently.

To many people in the West, acupuncture is a strange procedure, of which they are skeptical. It is an art and a science that has been practiced for thousands of years, however, and its effects and benefits are often not acknowledged by orthodox Western medicine.

Acupressure

Acupressure is a therapy that is similar to acupuncture in that it uses the same geography of meridians and acupuncture (or acupressure) points. Instead of using needles, however, hands or feet gently pressure the appropriate points. Acupressure relaxes tense muscles, improves blood circulation, and stimulates the body's ability to heal itself.

Acupressure, which predates acupuncture, was developed approximately five thousand years ago by the Chinese. They discovered that pressing certain points on the body not only relieved localized pain, but could affect other parts of the body and internal organs as well. Acupressure was increasingly disregarded, however, as the Chinese began to use needles to stimulate the acupressure points.

Acupressure points are illustrated on pages 384–387 at the back of the book. The descriptions of treatments for various conditions will refer to these diagrams and name the corresponding numbers that are relevant to use. For example, in treating migraine headaches, the text will read: "GB 20, located below the base of the skull in the hollows between the vertical neck muscles." Once you locate the point on yourself or the person you are treating, apply firm and steady pressure. It will take practice and experimentation to find the points and pressure that work for you.

Acupressure is not intended to cure serious illness or replace orthodox medical treatments for those illnesses. It can, however, increase relaxation, improve circulation, and ease pain, thereby maximizing health. Since it utilizes the same points as in acupuncture, specific *chi* or blood regulating or nourishing benefits associated with the points can be realized. It is an inexpensive and simple therapy to learn and one that, if practiced correctly, is entirely safe. Here are some tips to bear in mind when administering acupressure to yourself or others:

- Use only gentle pressure; it should not cause any pain.
- Since there are a number of acupoints that are forbidden during pregnancy, you should work on a pregnant woman only under the instruction of a qualified acupuncture or acupressure practitioner.
- Do not use acupressure on someone who is taking drugs or alcohol.
- Do not administer acupressure immediately after eating.
- It is best for the patient to sit or lie down, as he or she may feel drowsy during a procedure.

Movement and Meditation

Advocates of Oriental medicine also believe that you can heal yourself through the dedicated practice of different kinds of movement and meditation.

The martial arts are different forms of exercise that require and develop supreme control, discipline, and strength in the individual. A gentle martial art, tai chi chuan, can help a person develop inner strength and control. The Chinese believe that movement is essential for the human body. Tai chi chuan involves slow, deliberate movements, a sense of communion with nature, and concentration on finding one's *chi*. The philosophy is that if one can locate one's *chi* and learn how to use it, one can maintain good health. Some martial arts schools offer classes in tai chi chuan, and it is an exercise that requires many years of dedicated practice to develop fully.

Another form of meditation, called chi-gong, is also used to find one's *chi*. Chinese doctors believe that a ball of *chi* is located in the abdominal or pelvic region, and through meditation people can learn to move their *chi* to the appropriate areas of their body. The idea, again, is to learn to influence the flow of *chi* so as to maintain its balance in the body.

Even when you are working with a doctor or trying to heal yourself, all Oriental medicine seems to require willing and dedicated participation on your part. Oriental medicine has been practiced for thousands of years, and it is effective. Of course, as with any healing treatment, not all forms will work in every case or all of the time. Oriental medicine does seem to substantiate, however, the connection of the mental and physical. This belief is inherent in the Eastern philosophy of health, and it is utilized to treat illness and to maximize health.

HOMEOPATHY

Homeopathy is a system of health care and treatment that was developed in the 1800s by Dr. Samuel Hahnemann. The philosophy of homeopathy is holistic, viewing the individual as a totality of interdependent parts and working from the notion that the mental and physical realms are inseparable. Hahnemann believed that orthodox medicine was a system of "contraries," meaning that doctors treated the symptoms of an illness by using drugs that oppose, or suppress, them. He began to call conventional medicine *allopathic,* meaning "different" and "disease, suffering." Hahnemann recognized that removing or masking symptoms did not treat the underlying cause of the illness, which could, in effect, develop into a more serious condition.

In homeopathy, symptoms are seen as a healthy response of the body's defense mechanism. The vital force, or vital energy, acts to keep the body in balance. When the body is threatened by some harmful external influence, the vital force (or defense mechanism) produces symptoms in its struggle against the harmful agent. Therefore, to a homeopathic doctor, fever is a sign that the body is fighting illness. A cough, which an allopathic doctor would try to suppress with medication, is seen by the homeopath as the natural way to expel mucus from the body. Bear in mind that this does not mean you must suffer with coughing all day long. You can use herbal cough drops and drink teas with honey, for example, to soothe your throat. However, if you are not willing to endure some discomfort during your sickness, you should reassess whether natural medicine treatments are appropriate for you.

Believing that drug prescriptions for specific illnesses often were based on an inadequate understanding of the drugs and their effects, Hahnemann began to test, or "prove," drugs on healthy women and men, including himself, to determine their effects. He tested remedies on people rather than animals because he knew that people usually react differently than animals do. This human testing is possible because the homeopathic remedies are nontoxic. In more than two hundred years of using the homeopathic formulations, there has been no reported case of a permanent adverse reaction.

In his provings, Hahnemann discovered that each remedy induced particular symptoms in a healthy person. When that remedy was given to a sick person exhibiting those same symptoms, it helped cure the person. Based on this notion that like cures like, Hahnemann formulated the Law of Similars. It states that a substance causing certain symptoms in a healthy person can cure a sick person with the same symptoms. The theory behind the Law of Similars is that the body enlists its own energies to heal itself and defend against illness. If a substance that causes a similar response in terms of similar symptoms is administered, the body steps up its fight against it, thereby promoting cure.

In an attempt to lessen the initial aggravating effects that remedies sometimes had on patients, Hahnemann administered very small dosages. Ironically, he discovered that the smaller the dose, the more powerful the effect. This led him to develop the Law of Infinitesimals, which states that the smaller the dose, the more effective it is in stimulating the body to respond against the illness.

In order to prepare smaller and smaller doses, Hahnemann would put a substance through a series of dilutions. He would begin with the original substance, putting one part in nine parts of an 87 percent solution of alcohol and distilled water. He then subjected to *succussion,* or vigorously agitated, the vial by striking it one hundred times against a leather pad. Hahnemann believed that subjecting the substance to succussion activated the therapeutic potential of it. This first step yields a one-in-ten dilution, also indicated as a "1× dilution." Hahnemann would then take one part of this 1× dilution and put it in nine parts of diluent, subjecting it to succussion to yield a 2× dilution. This process, referred to as the Law of Potentization, could continue indefinitely, producing increasingly potent dosages.

Hahnemann believed in administering one homeopathic remedy at a time in order to establish its effects. He treated all patients as whole people, taking their symptoms as part of their whole being rather than treating them separately, and apart from the rest of the person. This method differs from orthodox medicine in which specialists treat specific illnesses and body parts, and patients often take many drugs simultaneously.

Homeopathy views health as a state of freedom and well-being on three interdependent levels: physical, emotional, and mental. The most serious symptoms usually affect the deeper parts of a person; therefore, it is most important to treat the mental state, then the emotional, and finally the physical. This is in keeping with the holistic view of natural medicine, which treats the entire person—physically and mentally. In other words, a homeopath would say that it is not enough to treat you for migraine headaches, because if the stressors producing the migraines are not addressed, the migraines will recur or other symptoms could develop.

The German homeopath, Constantine Hering, who emigrated to the United States in the 1830s, recorded the changes in posttreatment symptoms. Based on his findings that healing occurs from the inside out, he laid the groundwork for Hering's Law of Cure, which is recognized not only by homeopaths but by acupuncturists and psychotherapists as well.

Hering's Law states that cure occurs from within outward, from the most vital to the least important organs. The body deals with the most significant aspect of the condition first, shifting during treatment to the next most important aspect, and so on. For instance, healing is believed to be in progress—from the inside out—if your chest pains subside but a skin rash develops. During homeopathic treatment, your condition can change so that the same or other remedies may be needed to facilitate the entire process of cure.

Hering's Law further states that symptoms will appear and disappear in the reverse order in which they originally appeared. The patient may also reexperience symptoms from a past condition. According to Hering, healing often begins with the upper body parts and descends. Therefore, if chronic headaches subside but stiff fingers are felt, the homeopath might believe that healing is taking place, and gradually the fingers should return to normal. At times, healing may not follow the traditional pattern of Hering's Law, but as long as the patient feels stronger and is improved overall, it is safe to assume that the treatment is working.

Based on the order "first, do no harm," homeopathy is a safe and effective system of treating many common acute and chronic ailments. For a temporary, minor, self-limited illness or injury, you probably can treat yourself with homeopathic remedies after consulting with your doctor. You can obtain remedies from homeopathic pharmacists, or even from some drugstores or health-food stores. For a more chronic, persistent illness, you should consult a qualified homeopathic practitioner. Professional homeopathic medical doctors graduate from conventional four-year medical schools with a Doctor of Medicine (M.D.) degree and often complete postgraduate training in homeopathy to learn this holistic specialty. Homeopathic schools can be found worldwide, but to master the art and science of the system, physicians often learn from experienced homeopathic doctors. The fees charged by homeopaths vary, as does insurance coverage. Some states and insurance companies honor homeopathic treatment and some do not, and some will cover it only if it is performed by a licensed medical doctor.

HYDROTHERAPY

Sometimes the most obvious and simplest remedies are the ones most often overlooked. Consider water—it composes two thirds of our bodies and covers four-fifths of the earth's surface. Human beings can survive for weeks without food but only a few days without water. How can an element so common and abundant possibly be useful in healing?

The use that probably comes to mind first is the practice of swimming as physical therapy or bathing in a whirlpool to soothe sore muscles. But water has other healthful benefits as well, and in its various forms it can even be used to treat injuries and illnesses. It can work on the whole body, as in a bath, or on one area, as in the use of a compress. Water benefits the entire body by reenergizing it. Using a water therapy on one body part can also affect another beneficially, such as the use of a hot footbath to aid decongestion. Every organ and cell requires water, which helps nourish, detoxify, and maintain the right temperature of the body.

One of the earliest records of the therapeutic use of water dates back to the Greek god of medicine known as Aesculapius. At his temples, bathing and massage were used as a form of cure. Hippocrates also used water therapeutically. He advocated drinking water to alleviate fever, and he believed that baths could fight sickness. The Greek doctor Galen, who wrote Rome's outstanding medical text, also believed baths, both hot and cold, had beneficial effects, as did the Greek medical writer Celsus. Of course, this is true, because, in fact, one of the major reasons that health has increased over the ages is that sanitation and hygiene have improved.

In the eighteenth century, German, English, and Italian clergy revived the therapeutic use of water. In 1797, a Scottish doctor, James Currie, wrote a book called *Medical Reports on the Effects of Water, Cold and Warm, as a Remedy in Fever and Febrile Diseases*. In the early nineteenth century, Vincent Preissnitz, a Silesian farmer, reinvented water therapy using methods such as dousings, showers, immersions, and single and double compresses. His procedures spread to England, Germany, and Scandinavia, as well as the United States.

Later in the nineteenth century, Sebastian Kniepp adapted Preissnitz's techniques into his own theories of hydrotherapy. Kniepp, born in Bavaria in 1821, was a frail and sickly person. After reading a pamphlet about water cures, he decided to plunge into an icy cold river in the middle of winter with the hope that it would cure his ailments. Kniepp jumped into the river every day, and although it might seem absurd, he claimed that over time he became physically stronger. Along with Preissnitz's techniques, Kniepp claimed that walking in cold water or on wet grass was therapeutic.

Hydrotherapy is based on the law of action and reaction. If the skin is heated, either by a hot bath or compress, blood is immediately drawn to the surface and then returns to the deeper blood vessels. Likewise, cold water will drive blood away from the surface, but will cause a secondary effect of warmth as the blood returns to the tissues and vessels from which it was pushed away. This concept of immediate action followed by a secondary and more lasting reaction is a basic principle of hydrotherapy.

The different forms and temperatures of water have different physical and chemical effects on the body. Cold water is essentially restorative and reenergizing. It can reduce fever, act as a diuretic and anesthetic, alleviate pain, help relieve constipation, and eliminate toxins from the body. Ice and ice water can relieve the pain of burns, help control bleeding, and reduce swelling from injury. Warm water, in contrast, has a relaxing effect. Hot baths induce perspiration, which is essential in eliminating toxins from the body. Hot compresses and baths can reduce pain and inflammation, although cold water should be used for inflammation due to injury. This is important because hot water increases blood flow and would thereby increase inflammation in an injury. Alternating hot and cold baths can help increase circulation. Steam is a form of hydrotherapy that opens pores, increases perspiration, and sometimes alleviates chest congestion. Humidifying air is good for those who suffer from sinus conditions and airborne allergies.

Water has therapeutic uses when used internally or externally, at varying degrees of temperatures and pressures, and in its three forms: ice, liquid, or steam. Ice can be used as an anesthetic to chill the skin and dull pain. Boiling water is an antiseptic that can cleanse food and clothing. Hot compresses placed on the abdomen and herbal teas can work as antispasmodics to relieve cramps. If you need a diuretic, try drinking ice water or herbal tea or applying a hot, moist compress on your lower back; these all affect the kidneys to increase urine production. Colon irrigation, enemas, genital irrigation, the drinking of water, the taking of a sauna or hot baths all help to eliminate toxins. Drinking an emetic, such as salt water, can induce vomiting in order to expel certain poisonous substances. Finally, hot or cold baths or showers, whirlpools, and salt baths have a stimulating effect, while warm showers or herbal baths can act as a sedative.

Many different types of water application are used in hydrotherapy. Local heat can be achieved with a moist, hot compress or hot-water bottle; local cold requires a cold compress, frozen bandage, or ice pack or bag. A cold double compress is a cold compress covered with a dry cloth, such as wool or flannel, which creates internal heat. A pack is a larger form of the double compress, or it can be a clay, mustard, or flaxseed poultice. Alcohol, water, or witch hazel can be used in sponging, and you can achieve tonic friction by rubbing with a sponge or washcloth. Therapeutic showers can alternate between hot and cold, and the pressure of the shower can vary. Steam is therapeutic too, from a sauna, vaporizer, or humidifier.

One of the most common and most appreciated hydrotherapy techniques is the bath, a total immersion of either the body or a part of the body, such as hands, feet, arms, eyes, or fingers. Depending on the ailment you wish to treat, baths can be cold, tepid, or hot, can be long or short in duration, and can involve massage using a sponge, bath mitten, or loofah brush to create tonic friction. Baths can consist of plain water or contain salts, herbs, oatmeal, or mud. Following is a list of bath additives and their therapeutic benefits:

Apple cider vinegar: Fights fatigue; relieves sunburn and itchy skin.

Borax/cornstarch/bicarbonate of soda: Good antiseptic.

Bran: Softens skin, and relieves itchiness.

Chamomile: Soothes skin and opens pores; helps to relieve insomnia and digestive problems.

Dead Sea salts: Restores body after injury.

Epsom salts: Increases perspiration, relaxes muscles, and helps to relieve catarrh.

Fennel/nettle: Helps to rid skin of impurities.

Ginger powder: Relaxes muscles, tones skin, and increases circulation. (Use in small amounts as it is very powerful.)

Hayflower/oatstraw: Helps to rid skin of impurities.

Nutmeg: Increases perspiration.

Oatmeal: Good for skin problems, such as itchiness, hives, windburn, and sunburn.

Pine: Increases perspiration, softens skin, and relieves rashes.

Rosemary: Stimulates blood circulation.

Sage: Stimulates sweat glands.

Salt: Promotes a relaxing effect.

Sulfur: Good antiseptic and helps to rid skin of parasites; helps relieve acne.

It is easy and inexpensive to treat yourself to a wide variety of baths. Most of the listed herbs and preparations can be bought in drugstores, herbal pharmacies, health-food stores, or through catalogs. Remember to purchase them in small quantities since they lose their potency in approximately one year.

BOTANICAL MEDICINE

Botanical medicine, also referred to as herbalism, plant healing, physiomedicalism, medical herbalism, and phytotherapy, uses remedies made from plants called herbs. Whereas botanists define herbs as any plants that do not contain woody fibers, medicinal herbalists define them as any plant that has healing properties. Herbal remedies can also come from trees, ferns, seaweeds, or lichens, and herbalists will use whole plants, rather than isolating the principal active compounds from them. Whole plants contain proteins, enzymes, vitamins, minerals, and other trace elements that readily assimilate in the body. In fact, the three fatty acids essential for life—linoleic, linolenic, and arachidonic—are all found in plants. Botanical medicine is a safe and natural way to treat specific ailments and assist recuperation from illness in order to restore physiological balance.

The history of botanical medicine goes back through the ages, with "recipes" for herbal remedies being passed from generation to generation. Plants are natural agents of cure, and animals have an instinct for their curative powers. You've probably seen a dog nibble on grass. No, he doesn't think he's part goat—but he might have a bellyache and is eating the grass to aid his digestion. For centuries, Native Americans have chewed willow-tree bark to cure headaches. The bark contains salicylic acid, the active ingredient in aspirin.

Traditional herbal medicine originated in ancient times in India, China, and Egypt, with the earliest records appearing in Egypt and Assyria. Many of the plants listed in these and in Greek documents are still used today. Over time, herbalists have compiled classifications—descriptions of plants arranged according to their medicinal properties. Today, there are more than 750,000 plants in the world, and only a small percentage have been evaluated. The World Health Organization investigates and supports herbal medicine throughout the world in order to learn more about this natural method of healing.

Plants are used not only in botanical medicine but in allopathic medicine as well, and once served as the basis for nearly all drugs. In order to appreciate the benefits of botanical medicine, it is useful to look at how allopathy has used plants in preparing drugs.

Until the 1800s, most drugs were given by mouth in the form of ground leaves, roots, or flowers, or in teas, tinctures, or extracts. Doctors studied botany as a matter of course, and herbalists without medical training, particularly women, also flourished.

Prior to the 1800s, there was no standard clinical evidence on which doctors could base their selection of drugs for treatment. In 1803, a German pharmacist isolated morphine from opium, signifying the first time that a pure active principle had been obtained from a crude plant drug. With this pure form of morphine, doctors could give exact doses, knowing their effects. In the mid-nineteenth century, there was a push to isolate pure forms of active principles from medicinal plants. By 1870, caffeine had been isolated from coffee, nicotine from tobacco, and cocaine from coca.

These isolated compounds are generally more toxic than the whole plants from which they are derived. Scientists and doctors believed it was better to treat patients with the purified drug, and they disregarded other compounds in the plant. Herbalists, however, recognized that the whole plant has a different effect from the isolated substance since it contains many other vital ingredients that interact to give an overall effect.

Besides using isolated principles, chemists also experiment with molecules to synthesize new drugs. Their goal usually is to increase the potency and efficacy of the drug. More potent drugs can be risky, however, given that doctors often prescribe numerous medications simultaneously. And some drugs are so potent as to be addictive. Adverse drug reactions, or side effects, are the most common effects of iatrogenic (doctor-caused) illness.

Many commonly used drugs are derived from plants. For instance, digitoxin comes from foxglove *(Digitalis purpurea)* and is prescribed for heart failure; atropine is from deadly nightshade *(Atropa belladonna)* and dilates pupils; morphine comes from the opium poppy *(Papaver somniferum)* and is a powerful painkiller.

Herbalists may use the root, rhizome, stem, leaf, flower, seed, fruit, bark, wood, resin, or whole plant in preparing an herbal medication. Familiar with the interaction of various plants with each other, herbalists usually will use several plants or extracts in one preparation, since they can sometimes be more effective when combined than when used separately. Plants contain oils, alkaloids (nitrogen compounds), tannins, resins, fats, carbohydrates, proteins, and enzymes that all contribute to their medicinal action. Each substance has a function and can support, control, or otherwise affect the other constituents. In using the whole plant, the herbalist will get the most gentle, safe, and effective benefit from the treatment.

Herbal remedies can be taken in the form of tablets, capsules, lotions, ointments, suppositories, inhalants, or teas and juices. For herbal drinks, the basic proportion is 1 ounce (25 grams) herbs to 1 pint (0.5 liter) liquid. Herb teas will keep for three days in a tightly covered container in the refrigerator. Following is a list of common terms referring to botanical medications:

Carminative: Relieves flatulence, colic.

Cholagogue: Stimulates release of bile from the gallbladder.

Decoction: Drink made from roots, bark, or berries simmered in boiling water and strained.

Demulcent: Soothing substance for the skin.

Emmenagogue: Stimulates menstruation.

Emollient: Used internally to soothe membranes or externally to soften skin.

Infusion: Boiling water is poured over leaves, flowers, or the whole plant (excluding seeds and berries).

Nervine: That which is calming.

Ointments: Applied externally; effective for skin conditions.

Poultice: Crushed plant and hot water mixed to produce a paste that is wrapped in a thin cloth and applied to the skin.

Pressed juice: Juice from fresh plants is rich in vitamins and minerals; can be used in tinctures or diluted in water.

Teas: Made from pouring boiling water over fermented leaves or stalks from one or more plants; fermentation produces tannin; premade teabags can be purchased.

Tinctures: One part herb in five parts of diluted alcohol.

Tisane: Add boiling water to fresh or dried plant, usually green leaves.

You can dry your own leaves by laying them on a wire rack in a warm dry place for forty-eight hours; store in airtight glass containers. This should keep for one year. When preparing a tisane, use a separate pot from tea, as tannin will interfere with the tisane remedy.

Vulnerary: Used to treat and heal wounds.

An herbalist can give you information as to appropriate herbs used to treat various symptoms. A consultation with an herbalist is similar to one with other natural healers. The herbalist will check your heart and pulse, physical symptoms, and perhaps perform some laboratory tests, such as blood and urine analyses. More important, the herbal practitioner will spend quite some time observing, talking, questioning, and listening to you in order to determine the imbalance and disharmony of your body and life.

If you find a satisfactory course of treatment with a particular herbalist, it is good to stay with that person so as not to disrupt the healing process. Sometimes symptoms are aggravated before healing occurs, and some people and certain disorders take longer to heal than others. Patience and willing participation in your treatment is essential in order to maximize the benefits of botanical medicine. And any herbal treatment should be undertaken only in consultation with your physician.

PHYSICAL MEDICINE

Chiropractic

The word *chiropractic* means "treatment by the hands, or manipulation." It is a system of healing that was developed by David Daniel Palmer (1845–1913) in Iowa in 1895. Palmer believed that displacements of the spine caused pressure on nerves, which created pain or symptoms in other parts of the body.

Although chiropractic medicine subscribes to traditional concepts of anatomy and physiology, it differs from traditional medicine in that it is holistic, meaning it considers the patient as a whole, with an emphasis on body structure. Practitioners rely on X rays and standard orthopedic and neurological tests to diagnose problems, focusing on abnormalities of the spine. Treatment often involves direct thrust on specific vertebrae that are out of alignment, which helps to restore the flow of energy. Two terms that you will encounter in chiropractic are *adjustment* and *manipulation*. Adjustments involve dynamic thrusts (rapid, precise, and painless force) to a specific vertebra in order to remove any interference with nerves. It is not only the adjustment itself that is important, but the body's healing reaction to it. Manipulations are more general reorderings of bones to realign joints and increase the patient's range of motion.

Chiropractic is helpful in treating many conditions, including back pain and musculoskeletal disorders as well as certain systemic illnesses, such as asthma, migraines, and digestive problems. These systemic disorders, however, can be helped only if there is evidence of a structural and neurological involvement. Chiropractic treatment must be administered by a qualified and licensed professional, and it usually involves multiple visits in order to maintain proper spinal alignment. Initial visits can run from $50 to $150, with routine visits priced at approximately $50, and most insurance companies do provide coverage for this treatment. Chiropractors usually undergo at least two years of college plus an additional four years of professional education, and they must pass state and national licensing examinations.

Massage

The word *massage* derives from both the Greek *masso* ("knead") and the Arabic *mass* ("press gently"). It is a form of physical medicine that is completely harmless, comfortable, and relaxing. While a massage can be given by anyone, a trained massage therapist often seems to have a magic touch.

Massage works on the soft tissues, muscles, and ligaments of the body. It stimulates circulation and the function of the nervous system and helps to lower blood pressure. It can soothe muscle tension and headaches and can help relieve insomnia. Massage is particularly beneficial after exercise. During a workout, waste products build up in the muscles. It can take the lymphatic system days to wash them away. Massage speeds up this process by improving the circulation of blood and lymph.

There are two main types of massage: shiatsu and Swedish. Shiatsu was developed in Japan at about the same time that acupuncture began to flourish in China. This massage involves finger pressure that stimulates the acupuncture points along the body's meridians. One form of shiatsu firmly massages certain areas of the body to stimulate the flow of energy and restore balance. Another form involves the use of a single fingertip to stimulate acupuncture points. The purpose of shiatsu is to alter the flow of energy within the body, and it works along the same principle as acupuncture. Shiatsu therapists also emphasize the importance of good nutrition and positive mental outlook, and they encourage clients to make life-style changes that promote greater health. Shiatsu can be combined with chiropractic to maximize its healing effects.

Swedish massage, which is more common in the West, involves four essential techniques, with the underlying premise that the hands should not lose contact with the body. Swedish massage is effective because of its continual, rhythmic motions. These are the basic techniques.

Effleurage: Rhythmic stroking with open hands, with movements directed toward the heart; this motion soothes and relaxes the body.

Percussion: Brisk rhythmic movements with alternate hands that include cupping, hacking (with sides of hands), pummeling (with fists), clapping, and plucking; this stimulates the skin and circulation.

Petrissage: Deep movement that involves lifting, rolling, squeezing, and pressing the skin; this stimulates muscles and fatty tissues, stretching taut muscles to relax them.

Pressure: As the thumbs, fingertips, or heel of the hand make small, pressured circular movements, friction stimulates superficial tissue.

When you visit a massage therapist, he or she probably will not take a detailed physical history, but you should inform him or her of any pains, illnesses, injuries, or recent surgeries you have had. The therapist usually will begin with the feet or back and will allow you a few moments to get used to the sensation of being touched and kneaded. It should be a thoroughly pleasurable treat!

Sessions are usually one hour long and cost approximately $30 to $70. Therapeutic massage is covered by some insurance companies when it is required by a doctor for the treatment of a particular ailment or injury due to an automobile or work-related accident. Massage is generally entirely safe, but you should not use it if the following conditions exist:

- Infectious, open wounds or bruises
- Varicose veins
- Fever
- Inflamed joints or acute arthritis
- Thrombosis or phlebitis (could disturb blood clot)

Reflexology

Reflexology is a technique of deeply massaging the soles of the feet and hands in order to affect various parts of the body that are ailing. It was developed in China and India at the same time that acupuncture originated. Reflexology was brought to England in the twentieth century by Dr. William Fitzgerald, who called it zone therapy. In the United States Eunice Ingham developed Fitzgerald's teachings in the 1930s. Today, reflexology is growing in popularity, with schools located in Europe and the United States. Many practitioners of reflexology also perform chiropractic, osteopathy, and homeopathy.

Reflexology works on the premise that internal organs share the same nerve supplies as certain corresponding areas of the skin. Practitioners believe that the entire body is represented on the feet, primarily on the soles. By pressing the proper points on the feet, one can stimulate the organ associated with that point. These points are not the same as acupuncture points or meridians, many of which are not even represented on the feet.

During a reflexology session, the client will lie on a massage table while the practitioner feels the feet for granulelike substances deep within them. These "crystals" are actually waste deposits that build up in the nerve endings and capillaries and restrict the free flow of blood. The reflexology treatment breaks up the deposits so that they can be flushed from the body.

As the reflexologist "reads" the feet, he or she can determine which organs are affected. The patient will usually feel pain when a particular point is pressed, and sometimes in the corresponding organ or area of the body. The practitioner applies pressure with the edge of the thumb or finger and rotates it clockwise. The pressure is deep but should not be too painful. A session usually lasts from thirty to ninety minutes, and a client may require several sessions. Reflexology is beneficial for functional disorders that can be reversed, such as sinus problems, constipation, asthma, bladder problems, headaches, and stress.

PSYCHOTHERAPY

Psychotherapy, or "talk treatment," is an invaluable natural therapy for fostering and maintaining overall health. There has been much discussion about the mind/body connection. Although this has been an inherent part of holistic medicine throughout the world over time, orthodox Western medicine is realizing more and more the power of the mind and the importance of psychological treatments.

Mental health is important to physical health and vice versa. Emotional problems cause stress, which evokes physical symptoms and illness; physical illness, likewise, can cause a person to become depressed or lose energy and motivation. Doctors and patients are increasingly aware of the interplay of the mind and body and that in fact they may be inseparable, or one and the same.

Psychotherapy often requires you to talk about your feelings and problems, but it also can involve action, such as finding ways to alter your patterns of behavior. Treatment can be conducted on an individual basis between therapist and client, or it can be held within a group format. Group therapy allows clients to support and help each other, which can be just as valuable as receiving guidance from a therapist. People who seek out psychological treatment are not necessarily sick. They may simply be seeking greater understanding about themselves and their behavior.

There are many different kinds of psychotherapy, and some are more beneficial than others for treating particular disorders or problems. You may not hit upon the right therapy immediately, but don't give up. Success and progress in psychotherapy often take much time. If you really feel it's not working for you (and you've discussed this with the therapist), try a different therapist, and you might get better results. Psychotherapy, like many holistic, natural treatments, requires a willingness on the part of patients to be open to the treatment and to help themselves. You might go to a psychotherapist or counselor with the hope that the doctor will "cure" you. In fact, it takes work by both the therapist and the client in order for the treatment to be effective. The following sections list the major types of psychotherapy.

Supportive Psychotherapy

In this treatment, you can openly discuss your problems and feelings in a trusting, comfortable environment. The therapist should be a good listener who allows you the opportunity to vent your feelings, and who may make suggestions or point out insights that will give you a sense of support, without the feeling of being judged.

Exploratory Psychotherapy

This kind of treatment encourages you to explore your problems and issues, rather than just airing them. The therapist is usually active in the discussion and will let you know if you are avoiding a particular issue. Many healthy people pursue exploratory therapy as a way of learning more about themselves or to deal with a particular issue or aspect of their lives that they feel needs resolving or improvement.

Psychoanalysis

This treatment, which was originated by Sigmund Freud at the turn of the century, has taken a variety of forms. In classical psychoanalysis, you lie on a couch and talk freely about feelings, dreams, or whatever comes to mind. The psychoanalyst interprets what you say in terms of your childhood experiences and relationship with your parents. Psychoanalysis is usually intensive and long-term.

Other forms of psychoanalytic treatment focus on how your early emotional experiences have affected your current feelings and perceptions of yourself and relationships. This kind of therapy can help free you from pent-up or repressed childhood anger, frustration, hurt, and dependency. By working through these feelings, you will gain a greater sense of self-understanding and self-esteem.

Gestalt Therapy

Introduced in the United States by Fritz Perls in the 1950s, this "humanistic" therapy believes that the present moment, not the past, is most important, and that every person is responsible for his or her actions and has the ability to change them. In a session, if something from the past is bothersome, the therapist will help you bring it into the present. Gestalt therapists use many techniques to increase your awareness of yourself in the moment. For instance, if you are crying in a session, the therapist might ask you to speak to your tears. Merely talking about them promotes greater distancing between yourself and your emotions. Another Gestalt technique is for you to behave in a session opposite from the way you feel. For example, if you are very shy, the therapist might ask you to act like an outgoing person. Doing this will allow you to become aware of a part of yourself that exists but has remained undeveloped or repressed.

Behavioral Therapy

Behavioral therapists believe that all behavior is learned either through conditioning or the reinforcement of specific actions. For instance, if your mother taught you when you were growing up that all animals are dirty, you might develop a fear of animals, such as dogs. When the behavior you learned is negative or maladaptive, adverse psychological symptoms (in this example, a phobia) can result. Behavioral therapy can teach you new ways of behaving to help you live a more positive, happy, and productive life.

Behavioral therapy can resolve phobias, sexual dysfunction, inhibitions, and increase self-assertiveness. The therapist will help you learn new behaviors to replace those that are maladaptive. One method is called *operant conditioning,* by which new behaviors are rewarded and undesirable ones are ignored. In the *modeling* technique, the therapist "models," or displays for you to copy, the new behavior you are to practice. *Systemic desensitization* is a step-by-step process to help relieve specific fears or inhibitions.

Cognitive Therapy

This therapy was developed by American psychologist Aaron Beck in the 1960s. *Cognition* refers to a person's thinking, perception, and memory. If the therapist views your cognition as the cause of your emotional problems, the therapy will try to alter your perceptions and thoughts about yourself in order to alleviate the symptoms or problems. For example, if you were constantly denigrated by your father when you were growing up, chances are you developed a low self-esteem and often feel worthless. A cognitive therapist would point out evidence to the contrary, emphasizing your achievements that prove your self-worth.

Couples Therapy

Those who are married or involved in a serious intimate relationship know that even the best relationships require work. In couples therapy, you can visit a therapist either together or separately in order to understand and resolve tensions that exist within your relationship. Therapy can be useful to both heterosexual and homosexual couples.

Family Therapy

Families are intricate, dynamic networks that often require an objective outsider to help clear the air or resolve conflicts. When one or more family members has a problem, it often throws the entire unit into crisis, and this is when therapy can be beneficial. A family therapist is able to observe how the family operates together and can help the members understand not only how to deal with each other but their own roles within the family.

Just as it is important to find the right kind of therapy, it is equally important to build a good relationship with your therapist. As with other kinds of relationships, this can happen spontaneously, or it may take time. Within the emotional context of therapy, it is often difficult to discern how you feel about your therapist. Bear in mind that it is valid and important to discuss the feelings you have toward your therapist with him or her. This might reveal insight as to how you relate to others.

The different kinds of therapists are distinguished by their training. *Psychotherapist* is a general term that refers to anyone who practices psychotherapy. A *psychiatrist* is a medical doctor who is trained in psychotherapy and can prescribe drugs for treating mental disorders. A *clinical psychologist* holds a doctoral degree in psychology and has training in psychotherapy. He or she cannot prescribe medicine, and may specialize in a particular type of therapy, such as psychoanalytic, behavioral, and so on. A *psychoanalyst* is a psychiatrist or psychologist who is specially trained in psychoanalysis.

You can seek psychotherapy from a private therapist or from a mental health center or clinic. Fees vary according to the practitioner, though some are willing to use a sliding scale—that is, they will charge a fee based on your income and the amount you are able to afford. Some insurance policies provide a psychotherapy benefit, while others do not. If your policy does, find out whether there is a limit to the number of sessions or if there is a cap on the amount of coverage provided each year.

BIOFEEDBACK

Biofeedback probably presents the greatest evidence of the mind's influence over the body. In a healthy person, physiological functions are performed and regulated by the brain and central nervous system. The mind, however, often interferes, such as under conditions of stress that produce tension in the body. Biofeedback can teach the patient to intervene under these conditions in order to restore balanced functioning in the body.

Conscious control can affect many body functions that can be measured accurately and continuously, such as heart rate, skin temperature, blood pressure, muscle tension, and brain waves. The biofeedback equipment that measures these functions includes the electroencephalograph (EEG), which records nerve and brain waves, the electromyograph (EMG), which registers muscle tension, and the galvanic skin resistance instrument (GSR), which detects the electrical conductivity of the skin to record states of arousal, excitement, or nervousness.

When you are hooked up to these machines, they convey information to you through signals that can be recognized and interpreted easily. For instance, when the instrument detects muscle tension, a red light might go on or a certain sound might be emitted to signal what is happening to you internally. You then can use this information, in addition to certain relaxation and imagery techniques, to begin controlling the muscle tension. The techniques that are used in combination with the biofeedback equipment include relaxation and autosuggestion exercises, visual imagery, and meditation. For example, if the equipment signals that your heart rate is increasing, you can use imagery, by imagining a calm, peaceful place, or meditate through the repeating of a mantra in order to relax your mind and body. In biofeedback treatment, therefore, the patient is not the object of the therapy, he or she *becomes* the therapy itself.

There are many applications for biofeedback, including stress-related illness, neuromuscular problems, and personal growth and increased self-awareness. Biofeedback can be effective treatment for emotional or behavioral problems, such as anxiety, depression, phobias, insomnia, tension headaches, and bruxism (teeth-grinding). It also can be used to treat illnesses considered by some professionals to be psychosomatic such as asthma, ulcers, colitis, diarrhea, cardiac arrhythmia, hypertension, Raynaud's syndrome, and migraines. Biofeedback can help victims of stroke, cerebral palsy, and muscle spasms in some functions of the muscles and movement. Since biofeedback increases your recognition and understanding of your total mind-body functioning, it also can be beneficial in enhancing personal growth and self-awareness.

Many general and psychiatric hospitals have biofeedback clinics, and it is probably best to undergo treatments administered by a psychologist who is trained in biofeedback. A psychologist would be helpful in the process of developing greater self-awareness, and you might even consider combining biofeedback with psychotherapy.

When you begin biofeedback sessions, you should be informed about the equipment being used and the learning process and receive information about the muscles and the physiological functions involved in the treatment. Having this knowledge will help you to relax during the treatment and will probably enhance its success. Remember that while you must be an active participant in biofeedback, too much effort can produce unwanted stress. The key is to relax using meditation, imagery, and other techniques, in order to focus fully on your internal states.

Biofeedback training can last weeks, months, or years, depending on your problem. Most people need at least six weeks' worth of sessions, which last from thirty to sixty minutes and can occur once a week or daily, again, depending on the need. The cost of biofeedback varies depending on your location, with an average cost of $75.00 per session. Check your insurance plan for coverage. You must learn to transfer what you learn from the biofeedback sessions to your daily life. It will take practice to begin to recognize the signs of trouble—such as muscle tension, headaches, and so on—and the situations in which they occur, and then to use the techniques that can relieve them without the biofeedback instrument. You probably will need periodic checkups in order to maintain the progress you have made.

NUTRITION

The value of good nutrition may be obvious, but it is often the obvious that is overlooked. If you do not eat the right foods, the organs and cells of your body will not get the nutrients they need to function and grow properly. Since food is a basic necessity, it also has been looked upon as essential medicine from very early times. People in ancient Greece and Egypt, for example, used garlic as a cure for respiratory infections, intestinal viruses, and skin conditions. Cabbage was a remedy for ulcers and headaches. In the 1700s, English ships began to carry lemons and limes to treat scurvy, a condition that affected sailors.

It wasn't until the 1900s that scientists discovered the actual substance in citrus fruit that prevented scurvy. By this time, vitamin C had been isolated from lemons, and the first fat-soluble vitamin, A, was discovered.

By the 1940s, forty nutrients and thirteen vitamins had been isolated from foods. With the 1950s and 1960s came the era of processed foods, including the booming fast-food industry. This was followed in the next two decades by numerous fad diets as people desperately tried various ways to get rid of the weight gain that comes with this convenience.

Today, it seems that the public has a greater awareness of the kinds of things they ingest. New information on the dangers of substances such as pesticides, food additives, and saturated fats—and the benefits of nutrients—have altered the way many people eat. As you revamp your diet, however, it is important to read as much as you can in order to make informed choices about what you eat. Sometimes it is difficult to discern what is the latest fad and what is sound advice. Dieticians and nutritionists can help tailor your diet to your needs if you wish to pursue nutritional therapy to treat illness or allergies, or to bolster your health.

Essential Nutrients

All food is composed of certain substances that are necessary to maintain health: fats, proteins, carbohydrates, vitamins, minerals, and trace elements. Foods are characterized by categories (fat, carbohydrate, protein, dietary fiber), and a healthy diet balances a combination of them.

Protein   Approximately 17 percent of your body is composed of protein, including muscle, hair, bone, nails, and skin. Protein is also necessary for the production of hormones and enzymes. Since protein cannot be stored in the body, it must be absorbed regularly from foods such as milk, yogurt, cheese, eggs, meat, fish, sprouts, nuts, seeds, and legumes. If you do not eat enough protein, your muscles and tissues will degenerate. Too much protein, however, could strain the liver and kidneys and disrupts the balance of minerals in your body. Protein should account for approximately 5 percent of your total caloric intake each day.

Fats   Fat is an important source of energy. It helps to maintain organs, cell structure, nerves, and body temperature. Fat also carries fat-soluble vitamins, such as A, D, E, and K, around the body. There are three types of fatty acid: *saturated fat* primarily comes from animal sources, such as meat, fish, butter, cheese, eggs, and cream; *polyunsaturated fat* comes from plant sources, such as wheat germ and safflower, corn, and sunflower oils; *monounsaturated fat* is found in olive oil, avocados, and peanuts. Saturated fats, which can increase cholesterol levels, are the worst kind of fat to consume. Most people in our society would probably benefit from reducing their overall fat intake. Fat should constitute no more than 30 percent of your total daily caloric intake, with only 10 percent of this coming from saturated fats.

Carbohydrates   Our main source of energy is carbohydrates, which are converted into the glucose and glycogen that fuel muscles, the brain, and the nervous system. Carbohydrates come from starches and sugars. The best are starches in grains, legumes, and pastas, and sugars in fruit and vegetables. Refined sugar and flour contain high-calorie carbohydrates with little nutritional value. Unlike natural starches and sugars, which convert into glucose more slowly and are absorbed at a steady pace over time, they are absorbed quickly for instant bursts of energy. Carbohydrates should constitute the balance of your daily caloric intake (about 60 percent).

Dietary Fiber   Fiber, also referred to as roughage, is an indigestible substance found naturally in cereals, beans, nuts, vegetables, and fruits. Containing no nutrients and remaining undigested, it moves through the intestinal tract. As it absorbs liquid, it helps produce large soft stools that are easily passed. Fiber helps speed the passage of waste through the bowel and helps to remove toxic substances from the body. Low-fiber foods can take three or four days to pass through the digestive tract; high-fiber foods, in contrast, are usually passed within twenty-four hours. By consuming an adequate amount of fiber—and thus helping to move waste through the bowel more quickly—you may reduce your chances of developing colon cancer, diverticular disease, and gallstones.

Fiber occurs naturally in a wide variety of foods. Whole-grain cereals; whole-wheat, or bulgar-wheat, products; brown rice; barley; and bran are excellent sources of roughage. Legumes, oats, barley, and rye are also good sources and they form substances that restrict the amount of fat and sugar the body absorbs. This can help lower blood cholesterol levels and blood pressure. Corn, apples, carrots, brussels sprouts, eggplant, celery, potatoes, peas, and dried fruit are all good sources of dietary fiber. You should consume approximately one and one-half to two ounces (forty to sixty grams) of fiber each day.

Vitamins/Minerals   Vitamins and minerals are essential in aiding metabolism and the chemical processes in the body that release energy from food. The thirteen major vitamins are A, C, D, E, K, and eight B vitamins, often referred to as the B complex. Vitamins are soluble in either water or fat. Vitamin C and most of the B vitamins are water soluble. They must be consumed each day since they cannot be stored in the body. Any excess C or B vitamins are excreted. Vitamins A, D, E, and K are fat soluble, and they can be stored in the body's fatty tissues. Vitamin B_{12} can be stored in the liver.

Vitamins and minerals often work together and interact with each other. For example, vitamin C enhances the absorption of iron in the body. It is best to eat the daily required amounts of each vitamin and mineral in food.

If you decide to consult a nutritionist or dietician, he or she will help you devise a balanced diet and will recommend the supplements you should take according to any deficiencies you might have. If you are creating your own nutritional plan—or just modifying your eating habits—you should take a multivitamin and mineral supplement every day. This will ensure that you are getting the adequate amounts of nutrients that your body needs.

A Healthy Diet

Whole foods, or those produced with a minimal amount of processing, contain many of their original nutrients. Try to eat organically grown fruits and vegetables that have not been subject to chemical pesticides, meat and poultry that have not been given growth-hormone injections, and eggs from free-range chickens.

Generally, most people in our society need to eat more fruits and vegetables and to consume more fiber. It is best to eat fruits and vegetables raw and with their skins to ensure that you are getting all of their vitamins and minerals. Make sure to clean the skin thoroughly by scrubbing it with a brush (either a vegetable or pot-scrubbing brush) under running water to wash away unabsorbed chemicals from pesticides or other impurities. Fruits and vegetables should be eaten fresh, as they lose nutrients with age. They also lose nutrients through cooking, so try to cook them for as short a time and with as little liquid as possible. For example, if you usually boil vegetables, try steaming them instead. You'll probably enjoy their crispy texture and find that they have more taste! If you do boil your vegetables, consider using the liquid in stocks or sauces so as not to waste the vital nutrients.

Most of us also need to eat more fiber. If you now use white bread, try switching to whole-grain breads and cereals. Increase your fiber intake gradually in order to avoid a bloated feeling, which may occur temporarily.

If you want to consume less fat, eat only lean red meat in modest portions, and cook more poultry and fish. There are many good-quality low-fat products on the market, such as low-fat margarine. But use common sense in planning your diet. Remember that it is better to use just a little butter, a natural product, than to eat a lot of margarine, which contains added chemicals and hydrogenated fats. You also should consider using skim milk and low-fat yogurt and cheese. Avoid eating rich desserts, such as ice cream or pastries, fried foods, and rich sauces.

Most of us can probably do with less sugar and salt in our diets. Refined white sugar has no nutritional value, so try cutting down your use of it. If your sweet tooth will not be denied, replace sugar with honey or fruit juices—they are natural sweeteners. Try eating fruit or sugarless baked goods and jams that are sweetened only with fruit juices.

Although some salt is necessary, most people consume too much of it since it is used in excess in many processed foods. Remember, salt occurs naturally in many foods, so there is no reason to add more. Substitute herbs and spices for salt when you are cooking, and try to eat fewer processed foods. Generally, you should consume one ounce (twenty-five grams) or less of sugar and less than one-fourth ounce (six grams) of salt each day.

It was discovered long ago that honey and salt could help preserve foods. Over the past few decades, the use of artificial additives and preservatives has increased greatly, replacing the natural ones. Some of these are harmless in small amounts, and some additives even occur naturally, such as monosodium glutamate (MSG) in fermented soy products (soy sauce). However, when restaurants add excess amounts of MSG in the preparation of food, some people experience adverse physical symptoms, such as headaches, nausea, and dizziness.

Dyes, preservatives, stabilizers, antioxidants, and emulsifiers are all food additives that can cause reactions in people who are sensitive to these substances. Most additives are thoroughly tested for safety, and they must be listed on each product, according to the rules of the Food and Drug Administration (FDA). They are not all bad, but some people are particularly sensitive to them, and they can adversely affect hyperactive children.

In order to test your own sensitivity, or that of your child, to certain additives, you need to begin a very restricted diet of bland basic foods. Gradually reintroduce one at a time those foods that are suspect and record any reactions. It is best to consult a nutritionist, naturopath, or doctor who specializes in food sensitivities when conducting a test such as this.

The best advice for planning good nutrition is to avoid foods that you know you are allergic to and to maintain a balanced diet. Eat low-fat, high-fiber, naturally sweetened foods, and let moderation and common sense be your guide.

Calorie Chart

The word *calorie* refers to a unit of energy. Calories represent the amount of energy needed to burn a particular substance. The number of calories each person needs for maximum energy depends on age, sex, occupation, and lifestyle. The following chart serves as a guide for the amount of daily caloric intake for various groups of people:

MEN

Age	Lifestyle	Calories Needed Daily
18–35	Inactive	2,500
	Active	3,000
	Very active	3,500
36–70	Inactive	2,400
	Active	2,800
	Very active	3,400

WOMEN

Age	Lifestyle	Calories Needed Daily
18–55	Inactive	1,900
	Active	2,100
	Very active	2,500
56–70	Inactive	1,700
	Active	2,000

In their quest for health, fitness, and the perfect body, many people become almost obsessive about counting calories. Remember that it is not so much the number of calories you consume but where they come from that is important. In other words, it is better to eat 400 calories' worth of pasta and vegetables than of ice cream. The key to planning and following a healthy diet is balance. Eat a variety of whole foods from the basic food groups, and eliminate or moderate your consumption of those foods that you know are not good for you.

Orthomolecular Medicine

Ortho is the Greek word meaning "to correct." Two-time Nobel Prize winner Linus Pauling coined the term *orthomolecular medicine* in 1968 to refer to a system of correcting the body's metabolism with the right combination of nutrients, such as vitamins, minerals, amino acids, and enzymes. All of these nutrients occur naturally in the body as a defense against illness, but sometimes the body becomes deficient in one or many of them.

In 1943, the National Resource Council's Food and Nutrition Board established the Recommended Dietary Allowances (RDAs) of various nutrients. In 1963, the Food and Drug Administration created minimum daily requirements called U.S. RDAs, which are used by food manufacturers. The levels of U.S. RDAs are based on the lowest levels necessary to prevent known diseases, such as scurvy, which are caused by deficiencies. However, these levels are not necessarily high enough to promote health and combat other common illnesses. Orthomolecular doctors and other scientists advocate setting nutritional standards not based on avoiding diseases, such as scurvy, but on promoting optimum health.

Orthomolecular medicine is holistic in that it considers mental and physical causes of biochemical imbalances in the body. Practitioners perform blood tests and use vitamin and mineral profiles to delineate levels for sixteen vitamins and thirty minerals. Many physical and mental disorders can be treated simply by supplementing deficiencies in these nutrients.

Since each individual is unique, each has different nutritional needs. People who take megadoses of nutrients should take breaks from their dosages in order to prevent overdose. Orthomolecular treatments should be supervised by a trained doctor or nutritionist.

EXERCISE

Most of us live rather sedentary lives—we drive instead of walking or riding a bike; we sit at work; and we watch television while resting on the couch. Yet exercise is vital to our physical and emotional health. It improves muscle tone and posture, increases strength and stamina, and can improve circulation and respiration. Not only does exercise reduce blood-fat levels, it can change large blood-fat globules (low-density lipoproteins) to smaller, less sticky ones (high-density lipoproteins) that move more easily and are less likely to clog arteries. Exercise also is good for the mind. It invigorates and energizes, and helps to relieve tension and anxiety. By helping to release substances that affect emotions, such as adrenaline and noradrenaline, exercise can even relieve the symptoms of depression. Have you ever heard of a runner's high? The explanation for runners' "addiction" to their exercise is that it helps to release endorphins and enkephalins, which have a mood-elevating effect. When you exercise, your body gets in shape and your mind begins to relax.

There are several different kinds of exercise, and a good workout routine should include a little of each. *Isotonic* exercises, such as weight training, stretching, and yoga, develop muscle strength and flexibility. They do not have the aerobic benefits of improving respiration and circulation, but they are essential for toning slack muscles and building strength. *Stretching* exercises, as part of your warmup and cool-down, are a must in any kind of workout.

Aerobics refer to sustained exercise that increases the amount of oxygenated blood carried to muscles and organs. In other words, any activity that increases your breathing and heart rate is aerobic: aerobic dance, step aerobics, running, jogging, fitness walking, cycling, swimming, and cross-country skiing. Stationary bicycles, Lifecycles, and StairMasters are aerobic fitness machines. When you perform an aerobic exercise, you should maintain your training-level heart rate for fifteen minutes or longer in order to receive maximum results. (See the chart on p. 66.) Aerobic exercise improves the respiratory and circulatory systems. It strengthens the heart muscle, makes arteries and veins more elastic, and lowers blood-fat and body-fat levels.

Anaerobic exercise is the opposite of aerobic exercise. It is characterized by short bursts of energy, such as sprinting. Although anaerobic exercise does develop muscle strength, it does not improve circulation and respiration.

When you plan an exercise regimen, consider activities that you enjoy, that are feasible, and that you will want to do. That way you'll have a better chance of maintaining your exercise routine. Some people like to exercise alone —it is "quiet" time to think or clear the mind. Others prefer to exercise with a partner or a group because other people can be a good source of motivation and can make exercise a fun social event. You also need to consider how much time you can allot to the activity. When you have a very busy schedule, it is easy to forgo the exercising, especially if you are tired. Just try to remember that the more you do it, the more energy you will have in the long run for all of your life's activities.

If you are over the age of forty and have been relatively inactive, are pregnant, or have another medical condition, you should consult a physician and have a complete physical exam before beginning an exercise program. When you start, begin slowly and gradually increase the duration and intensity of your workouts. Warming up is a must—stretch your muscles slowly and smoothly for at least five minutes. The endurance phase of your workout should last approximately twenty to thirty minutes, getting your pulse rate up to training level. Cooling down is also imperative—spend five to ten minutes walking briskly and doing more stretching exercises.

The following chart will help you determine your training-level pulse rate. The resting pulse of adults is generally sixty to eighty beats per minute. To take your pulse, use the first three fingers of your hand to feel the beat in your temple or neck. Count the number of beats in fifteen seconds and multiply that by four to equal one minute.

Age	Beats per minute for Training Level
20	138–158
25	137–156
30	135–154
35	134–153
40	132–151
45	131–150
50	129–147
55	127–146
60	126–144
65	125–142
70	123–141
75	122–139
80	120–138
85	119–136

Once you get into the swing of an exercise routine, you'll probably look forward to the activities—and even feel bad if you skip a session. Remember to use common sense when you are exercising, especially if you do strenuous aerobic activity. Here are some tips:

- Do not exercise if you are ill, dizzy, or feel faint. If any of these feelings occur during a workout, cool down by walking and stretching, and then take off a day or two.
- Do not exercise if you feel severe muscle or joint pain; take a few days off and begin again gradually. If pain persists, consult a physician.
- Always warm up and cool down to avoid stiff or injured muscles.
- Allow two hours after meals before exercising.
- Avoid exercising in very hot weather and dress warmly in cold weather if you exercise outside; even if you perspire, keep all of your clothing on to avoid chilled muscles that can result in cramps or pulls.
- "No pain, no gain" may be true to a degree, but you should build the intensity of your workout gradually. Use common sense, listen to your body and mind, and don't overdo it!

CHAPTER THREE

A First Look at Asthma and Allergy

Does it seem as though more and more people are complaining about allergies? Are you finding yourself allergic to substances that didn't bother you at all in the past, or are your allergies changing, maybe even becoming worse? And are you having new, or increased, asthma symptoms? Individual genetics, age, and overall health combine to create your own unique allergic makeup. But advances in modern medicine and technology, and the environment, may also be conspiring against us.

Medical advances during the past century have provided us with an array of lifesaving medicines, such as antibiotics and insulin. These medicines save lives, but at the same time, they have the potential to alter the immune system, which is where allergies begin. We are also eating more chemicals, from the pesticides sprayed on plants to the preservatives lurking in prepared foods. We're breathing polluted air, which can lead to or exacerbate asthma. And while a century ago you were likely to have spent your time close to home, you can now hop on a plane and send yourself to the other side of the world within a matter of hours. With travel comes exposure to even more allergens. Furthermore, air conditioning recycles bad air throughout the buildings we work and live in.

The relationship between the environment and allergy is complicated, and scientists are still learning about the cause-and-effect nature of this relationship. However, environmental factors can certainly trigger responses in the immune system, which can include asthma and allergy.

Regardless of the kinds of allergy symptoms you experience, allergic reactions begin in the immune system. The immune system is the first line of defense against foreign invaders, and its job is to be on the lookout for germs and viruses, and to destroy them.

ALLERGY'S ROOTS: THE IMMUNE SYSTEM

The immune system is a related set of responses, spread throughout tissues of various organs in your body. It consists of free cells, called lymphocytes, which manufacture and secrete molecules called antibodies. And these antibody molecules are not all identical. They are structured to recognize and attack various antigens, with patterns that distinguish one type of molecule, such as a protein, from bacteria and viruses. Generally, the human body does not attack its own molecules.

Lymphocytes and antibodies are carried by the bloodstream into all the organs, and then return to the bloodstream through the lymphatic system. These lymphocytes accumulate in lymph nodes, located at various sites throughout the body. Additionally, the bone marrow, the thymus, and the spleen are also attached to the lymphatic system.

When a potential invasive element, like germs or bacteria, is detected by the immune system, organs or glands such as the lymph nodes produce cells that attach themselves to these elements and neutralize them. For example, T cells actually attach themselves to the invasive element, and attack it while the B cells produce antibodies. This immune system reaction can keep you from developing a serious infection.

The human body continually learns to protect itself from disease. Once it has produced an antibody to a specific antigen, such as a virus, it continues producing that antibody in addition to others. Through vaccination, antibodies are introduced into the system to prevent an illness such as measles.

Allergens Enter the Scene

While antibodies provide protection, your system can also produce antibodies to protect you from molecules that you don't necessarily need to be protected from. For individuals who are allergy prone, exposure to substances known as allergens, such as pollen, dust, insect venom, or certain foods, can result in production or overproduction of an antibody.

While the number of potential allergens is almost infinite—and you may have a long list of your own—they tend to fall into the following groups:

Animal dander and saliva
Cleaning products
Cold temperature
Cosmetics
Drugs
Dust
Fabric
Feathers
Foods
Fur
Insect venom

Molds and fungi
Perfume
Poisonous plants
Pollen
Solvents
Tobacco smoke

As you look through this list, you may recognize some of your own allergies, or a few that you haven't considered before. Also notice that contact with some of these allergens is through inhaling. Others are eaten, touched, or injected.

Immunity Run Amok

When an allergy-prone individual is exposed to an allergen, his or her body reacts by producing antibodies called immunoglobulin E, or IgE. Each IgE antibody is specific for one particular allergenic substance. For example, if you have an allergy to pollen, your body actually produces one antibody for each specific type of pollen, that is, one for ragweed and another for oak.

These IgE molecules attach themselves to the body's mast (tissue) cells, and white blood cells, called basophils. When the allergen next encounters the IgE, it attaches to the antibody like a key fitting into a lock. This signals the cell to which the IgE is attached to release powerful inflammatory chemicals like histamine, prostaglandins, and leukotrienes. These chemicals move into various parts of the body, such as the respiratory system, the skin, or the gastrointestinal system, and cause the symptoms of allergy.

Here's more on how it works. Allergic reactions result from the body recognizing a common substance, such as cat hair, as an allergen and therefore an enemy, and trying to protect itself with the production of antibodies. Thus, allergies are an immune system response that has gone out of control—run amok. When the immune system has produced enough antibodies against the allergen, a chemical called histamine is produced. Normally, histamine stays inside the cells and is not a harmful substance. However, when released outside of the cells, and circulated through the body, it causes some of the blood vessels to constrict and others to dilate. When the blood vessels dilate, the fluid from the blood vessels leaks into the tissues. Histamine causes discomfort in whatever area of the body it is released.

For hay fever sufferers, histamine is released in the nasal passages, and the resulting symptoms include sneezing and congestion. Histamine in the brain causes headaches. If the histamine is released in the airways, the lining of the bronchial tubes may swell, a thick mucus is produced, and the tubes may even close. This is what happens in an asthma attack. Histamine in the digestive system causes stomach cramps and diarrhea, and in the skin, rashes or hives.

Allergic reactions are not always predictable; an allergic individual may at first have no reaction to an allergen, and then begin experiencing violent reactions at a later time. One reason for this lack of predictability is that a sufficient number of antibodies have to be produced by the immune system before histamine is even released, and the immune system generally has to be exposed more than once for the antibodies to be produced. While the results of histamine production can be predicted, as described above, the actual severity of an allergic reaction is not so simple to predict. It depends on factors such as state of mind, diminished body resistance, and hormonal changes. Furthermore, while scientists understand how allergies manifest themselves, they don't really know why some people have allergies and others don't. As you'll see later, genetics may play a role, as does the environment.

Regardless of how you actually come into contact with what, for you, is an allergen, the result is a set of physical symptoms called an allergic reaction. Suppose you have an allergy to cats, and you walk into a room and discover a cat sitting a few feet away from you. Chances are your reaction will be immediate, with symptoms such as sneezing, wheezing, sniffing, or a rash. Symptoms that appear so immediately constitute an anaphylactic reaction. A severe anaphylactic reaction, if not treated, can result in blocked airways, choking, heart failure, and even death.

AN OVERVIEW OF
ALLERGIES AND ASTHMA

Specific aspects of allergy and asthma, and treatment alternatives, are discussed in Chapters 4 through 11. To introduce you, here is an overview.

Food Allergy

Allergic reactions to food have always been somewhat of a mystery, both to sufferers as well as the practitioners who treat them. There simply doesn't seem to be an explanation for the unpredictable, though sometimes violent, symptoms of an allergic reaction to food.

The symptoms of an allergic reaction are also difficult to categorize and predict. For example, a food allergy sufferer who comes into contact with the offending food may experience an upset stomach, nausea, vomiting, and diarrhea. However, these same symptoms can also be caused by stress, as well as by food poisoning. As a result, treating food allergies requires extensive cooperation between the patient and the practitioner, with both willing to undertake what may seem like a very painstaking, methodical process to uncover the specific food allergies.

Skin Allergy

Allergies of the skin generally fall into three categories: rashes and hives, eczema, and contact dermatitis. Skin allergy reactions can result from exposure to plants, chemicals, cosmetics, lotions, or a wide range of other possible substances. A skin allergy can show up immediately—large red blotches on your hand, for example, or oozing bumps —or it can appear a day or two after exposure to the allergen. The symptoms can disappear just as quickly, or torment you for years.

Hives appear as raised red welts. Eczema, which is more commonly associated with children, and contact dermatitis, with adults, has symptoms that include redness, swelling, itching, oozing, and scaling.

Allergic Rhinitis and Hay Fever

The term "allergic rhinitis" refers to irritations of the nose that are caused by allergens. Allergic rhinitis is often used interchangeably with the term "hay fever," which refers to allergies that are caused by pollen. Hay fever sufferers, of which there are multitudes, generally suffer the most during spring, summer, and autumn when pollen production is at peak levels. During the fall, the mold spores produced by wet fallen leaves can also be irritating to hay fever sufferers.

The symptoms of allergic rhinitis and hay fever are the same. They include sneezing, watery nasal discharge, itchy soft palate, postnasal drip, occasional coughing, laryngitis, and teary eyes. Also, swollen nasal passages can lead to congestion that blocks the sinusus and keeps the mucus from draining, leading to sinus headache.

Year-round allergies are not necessarily the result of coming into contact with pollen. Air conditioners can circulate mold spores through the air. Forced heating systems also circulate mold and house dust. Allergic rhinitis sufferers may also be allergic to the fur and feathers of animals and the feathers in pillows and upholstery.

Asthma

Asthma is a very complex disease. While it usually starts in childhood, it can persist into adulthood, or even subside in intensity during adolescence only to return a few years later.

Symptoms include shortness of breath, coughing, wheezing, and some chest tightness. For some people, asthma symptoms occur rarely, while others suffer continuously. The conditions that bring about asthma symptoms vary greatly among individuals. Potential triggers include exercise, foods, tobacco smoke, a cold, a sensitivity to air pollution, or allergens including house dust, fungus, spores, pollen, and animal dander.

While allergies can affect many parts of the body, asthma affects the lungs. Though clinicians are not sure why, the bronchial airways of asthma sufferers tend to constrict more easily and quickly than normal. They become narrow, and this restricts air flow. The result of this constriction is an asthma "attack" with breathing difficulties and wheezing.

Asthma symptoms can be relatively light, causing some minor discomfort. But they can also be severe, even life threatening.

CAUSES OF ASTHMA AND ALLERGIES

No one really knows what causes allergy, and why allergic response patterns in one person differ so much from those of another. Asthma is equally mysterious, especially when symptoms appear for a few years, disappear, and then reappear during adulthood. Natural medicine views allergy and asthma as resulting from a range of factors, all interacting together. While conventional medicine focuses on factors like heredity, natural medicine practitioners look both to and beyond the realm of physiology, to factors like the environment and spirituality.

Heredity

Heredity is most certainly a factor in allergy and asthma, though how much of a factor depends on the individual. Did one of your parents, or maybe an uncle, suffer from allergy? If so, are you allergic to the same substances as your relatives, or to different ones? Like your eye color and height, the tendency to become allergic is an inherited characteristic. Yet, although you may be born with the genetic predisposition to become allergic, you will not be automatically allergic to specific allergens. Other factors must also be present for allergic sensitivity to be developed. The same is true for asthma. These factors include:

- The specific genes acquired from your parents
- The exposure to one or more allergens to which you have a genetically programmed response
- The degree and length of exposure

A baby born with the tendency to become allergic to cow's milk, for example, may show allergic symptoms several months after birth. A genetic predisposition to become allergic to cat dander may take three to four years of cat exposure before the person shows symptoms, that is, if the allergy is going to show up at all. These people may also become allergic to other environmental substances with age, or again, they may not. It is also possible to develop allergies with no known family history of allergy.

Environment

Environmental pollutants are recognized as playing a role in a range of illnesses, including cancer. While their role in allergy and asthma is not completely understood, pollutants do appear to contribute to both the development of allergy as well as the onset of an attack of symptoms. As a result of constantly breathing high levels of air pollution, the overall health of the lungs can be diminished, much the same as results from breathing tobacco smoke. The lungs are thus much more sensitive to allergens, as well as more prone to asthma and illnesses like bronchitis.

Diet

A poor diet, lacking in a balance of foods from the major food groups, also leaves the body susceptible to illness. Many natural medicine practitioners believe that a diet high in animal fats will contribute to the development of allergy and asthma, as does a diet high in food additives, such as preservatives and dyes. Natural medicine practitioners will often make diet recommendations as part of their treatment.

Emotions

For many allergy sufferers, there is a direct connection between emotional well-being and susceptibility to allergens. Stress sets your immune system on edge, which can lead you to react, and overreact, to allergens. And stress is a vicious circle: once your symptoms begin, fear and anxiety sensitize your immune system even more, and your symptoms can worsen. Natural medicine alternatives that deal with your emotional side, like meditation and psychotherapy, promote relaxation and emotional balance that can, in turn, reduce your allergy and asthma symptoms.

Spirituality

The connection among body, mind, and spirit is receiving increasing attention in our society. Yet while the relationship between the body and the mind seems relatively logical, the spirit remains a mystery. The definition of "higher power" is really up to each individual, though connection with a higher power results in feelings of centeredness and calm, and can add meaning to life. Your higher power can be God, Buddha, a spirit guide, your inner self, the universe, or whatever concept is meaningful for you. Some people believe that being out of communication with a higher power can leave you open to illness, while good health is the result of a unity among the mind, body, and spirit. Many natural medicine alternatives, including macrobiotics and visualization, promote spiritual health.

This comprehensive approach to understanding the roots of asthma and allergy is also reflected in the ways natural medicine treats asthma and allergy.

MAJOR NATURAL TREATMENTS FOR ALLERGY AND ASTHMA

Throughout the chapters that follow, you'll be presented with natural methods of treating your allergy and asthma symptoms. Some of these methods will help you relieve your symptoms; others will be useful in helping to prevent flare-ups of symptoms. Those that you will see most often are described in the following pages.

Acupuncture

Chinese medicine is based upon the belief in a universal energy that flows through all of nature, including the human body. This universal energy is called *chi,* which is sometimes spelled *qi* or *ki.* When this energy is balanced, flowing smoothly throughout the body, the result is good health. When the *chi* is blocked somewhere in the body, and therefore unbalanced, the result is illness. Energy flows along pathways, or meridians, with each of the pathways flowing through the organs of the body. These organs are not identical to Western organs. They have a wider energetic network associated with them.

Allergy and asthma, based on this philosophy, are the result of an imbalance of *chi.* In the case of allergy, this imbalance may lead to oversensitivity to substances like pollen, and a range of symptoms. The causes of these imbalances differ among individuals; there are no standard answers. Causes include stress, diet, lack of exercise, as well as a range of other possibilities.

As a branch of Chinese medicine, acupuncture is holistic in its approach. Acupuncture involves the use of very fine needles that are inserted at various positions in the meridians to restore the flow of energy. Rather than treating illness and specific symptoms, the goal of acupuncture is to restore energetic balance to the body. When the various organs and systems are back in harmony, illness disappears. For example, when an acupuncturist detects wheezing and difficulty in breathing, the various signs and symptoms would have to be differentiated to determine whether they resulted from an excess or deficiency of energy, and what energetic networks of the body were involved. A medical doctor, on the other hand, would probably diagnose the condition as asthma and begin to prescribe medications, without a differentiation.

While acupuncture is useful for treating specific conditions, it is also useful for reducing the effects of stress. As such it may be useful in preventing the onset of allergy and asthma symptoms. Often the treatment of asthma and allergies is most effective when targeted to the season *before* symptoms are usually at their worse.

Diagnosis: The Key to Treatment There are no quick and easy diagnoses in acupuncture because each patient is viewed as an individual, not simply as a set of symptoms. Thus, while illness is viewed as being caused by blocked energy, these blockages can be the result of causes that are not only physical but psychological. An increase in asthma or allergy symptoms, for example, can be the result of a breakup of a relationship that has allowed grief to injure the lungs. This is because each organ in Chinese medicine is associated with a specific emotion. Disease can result from an emotional imbalance, and imbalance in an organ can lead to emotional imbalance as well. The emotions cause *chi* to flow in certain specific ways. For example, in anger, *chi* rises to the head and shoulders, while in fear, *chi* descends to the feet.

Acupuncturists work for years to develop their diagnostic skills, learning to treat the whole person by relying on a range of components. When making a diagnosis the acupuncturist is seeking clues to the imbalances that may exist and, once the diagnosis is made, will begin to treat these imbalances. Thus, the diagnostic process will be the same for an individual complaining of allergy or asthma as it would be for someone with symptoms of back pain or anxiety. Depending upon the training of the acupuncturist, the most important aspects of diagnosis are the pulse and tongue, and palpation of meridians.

Pulse Traditionally, feeling the pulse has been one of the primary techniques of the acupuncturist, especially for those trained in Chinese styles of acupuncture. Other forms of training use the pulse only as a confirmation of other diagnostic techniques. Some acupuncturists (especially those who are more meridian and palpatory oriented) may not use the pulse at all. Rather than merely feeling for a few seconds and calculating the rate, as in Western medicine, acupuncturists feel the pulse in three different positions of the arm, using two different pressures on each pulse to learn something about each of the meridians. Not only does the acupuncturist count the pulses, but also ascertains how each one actually feels. What he or she seeks to determine is the nature of the energy in the body and where it is in balance, and where it may be in excess or deficient.

Tongue Along with the pulse, the acupuncturist also focuses on the tongue in making a diagnosis. In examining the tongue, the practitioner looks at the color to check for excesses or deficiency of yang or yin (described in Chapter 2). Conditions such as swelling, or a coating, depending on its color, will also tell the acupuncturist something about the balance of energy. Additionally, areas of the tongue correspond to major organs of the body, such as the stomach and gallbladder, and abnormalities of the tongue may indicate energy imbalances in one of these organs.

While examinations of the pulse and the tongue are the classical tools that the acupuncturist may use in making a diagnosis, other factors are also important. These are described below.

Palpation/Touch   The acupuncturist has a refined sense of touch, and is able to discern imbalances by palpating the course of a meridian. In addition, the acupuncturist may palpate your *hara*—the area from your pubic bone up to your rib cage—looking for areas of congestion, or deficiency, warm or cool spots, et cetera. This will give the acupuncturist detailed information about the energetic imbalances in your body, and selection of acupuncture points may be based on this information.

Facial Color   When the *chi,* or energy, is unbalanced, color changes may show up in the face. Turning pale or red are more obvious examples. However, an acupuncturist is trained to look for more subtle changes, especially around the mouth and on the temples.

Odor   Energy imbalances can also cause specific body odors. Fever, for example, can change the odor of the sweat. But many people have particular odors (e.g., sweet, burnt, et cetera) which are associated with particular energetic imbalances.

Taste   The preference for different tastes, such as sweet, spicy, or sour flavors, may change just as a result of imbalances, and the pattern of these changes is useful in determining the source of the imbalance.

Emotion and Tone of Voice Emotional imbalance often reveals itself in one's tone of voice. Acupuncturists learn to discern the tone of a client's voice and use it to diagnose a client's emotional constitution or acute imbalance.

Acupuncturists also observe other factors to diagnose what may be causing your asthma and allergy symptoms. These factors include your overall spiritual condition, the effect of the climate on your symptoms, the times of day when you are most and least energetic, and the seasons and temperatures in which you are most comfortable. In contrast to Western medicine, in Oriental medicine one disease may have many patterns of disharmony, and therefore many different treatments. For example, three patients with asthma may have three different energetic imbalances.

The Role of Symptoms Clearly, the kinds of symptoms you have can indicate the nature of your problem. Chest congestion points to problems in the lungs, but the congestion may stem from an imbalance in the spleen/stomach energies, resulting in too much phlegm. However, an acupuncturist will look beyond the obvious to other underlying causes. For example, while your lungs may indeed be malfunctioning, it may be the result of an energy imbalance in yet another organ. In other words, think of your body as a homeostatic balance, with a change in one sphere affecting other spheres.

Allergy and asthma symptoms can be the result of organs that are seemingly unrelated to the condition in Western terms. Most likely, your symptoms are the result of imbalances affecting multiple spheres. How these imbalances came about in the first place is the result of many different factors. Heredity comes into play. Emotions, not only those being expressed, but also those that may be repressed, like anger, can lead to imbalances. Toxins added to your system from the environment and the food you eat will further add to imbalances.

An acupuncturist will also listen to what you have to say about your symptoms. Questions an acupuncturist might ask include:

Is it more difficult to inhale or exhale?

Does the tightness you feel extend vertically down the center of your chest, or more horizontally across the top of your chest?

In what season are your symptoms worse?

Do you find that your symptoms are worse when you are under stress? What kind of stress?

Answers to these questions help the acupuncturist to discriminate among different patterns of imbalance.

After looking at this wide array of indicators, from the pulse to the tongue to the emotions, the acupuncturist makes a diagnosis of the most likely causes of your symptoms, and begins a course of treatment.

Treating Your Asthma and Allergy with Acupuncture Acupuncture is as much an art as it is a science. The practitioner's initial approach to treatment is based both on experience and intuition. If your symptoms are debilitating—difficulty in breathing, for example, excessive congestion, or eczema—and causing you discomfort, the practitioner might start out by focusing on providing immediate relief for your symptoms. This approach is based on one of the tenets of Oriental medicine: in acute situations, first treat the branch. In chronic conditions, treat the root of the problem.

In acupuncture, diagnosis is an ongoing process. Symptoms may improve, but the underlying conditions must also be improving. Your practitioner may determine this by checking your pulse, tongue, and other signs, and using palpation. If improvement is not occurring, the approach will be adjusted.

Aromatherapy

Aromatherapy—using essential oils for healing—has been around for thousands of years, though interest has increased over the last few years as individuals have become drawn to the benefits of natural health. Aromatherapy is a holistic approach to health, revolving around the administration of essential oils that promote the body's own natural healing abilities.

The oils used in aromatherapy are taken from the scent globules of plants. Scent globules are found in various parts of plants. These parts, and examples of the scents they produce, are as follows:

Flowers—chamomile, rose, and jasmine

Leaves—balm, sage, and thyme

Roots—vetiver and angelica

Fruit and seeds—coriander, caraway, and anise

Woody portion—cedarwood, sandalwood, and rosewood

Bark—cinnamon

Resin (used for incense)—benzoin, myrrh, and sandalwood

Fruit skin—orange, lemon, and bergamot

A skilled aromatherapist is trained to use distilled essences effectively in treatment. These essential oils are believed to contain a life force that carries energy that can be administered to humans and thus promote healing. No two plant types are alike in terms of their aroma or essence. As a result, each essential plant oil, such as jasmine, rose, and sandalwood, has unique properties, and is used for healing specific ailments.

As implied by the word *aroma,* aromatherapy involves the sense of smell. There is a scientific basis for this treatment. Fragrance molecules reach the brain during the breathing process, beginning with the olfactory bulb, which is located above and on either side of the inner nasal cavity. The olfactory bulb, called the olfactory epithelium, is lined with tiny olfactory nerve cells covered with a thin layer of mucus. Each nerve cell, which is replaced monthly, contains microscopic hairs, called cilia, that act as receptors. The cells in the olfactory membrane are brain cells, and through the olfactory membrane, the central nervous system is directly exposed to the environment. Every time you breathe, you are taking in information about your environment.

While scientists are unsure of how this whole process actually works, they do know that the sense of smell requires the presence of odor molecules. These molecules register in the brain, during the process of breathing, by stimulating the cilia in the olfactory nerve cells. As a result, while you may not yet be aware of the origin of a specific odor, the subconscious part of your mind is alerted to its presence and reacts accordingly. The result can be illness, as in an allergic reaction, or positive energy. The purpose of aromatherapy is to introduce this positive energy to your system.

The stimuli introduced to your central nervous system, through odors, result in the release of neurotransmitters. These neurotransmitters in turn can produce effects such as pain reduction and a sense of well-being. Serotonin, one of the neurotransmitters, results in a feeling of relaxation, while endorphins can stimulate sexual feelings. It all depends on the specific odor that has been introduced.

And here is the key to how aromatherapy can help you with allergy relief: While you can breathe in allergens that result in allergic rhinitis and hay fever reactions, you can also breathe in relief by using aromatherapy techniques.

Applying Aromatherapy   The best way to get started in applying aromatherapy is to locate a qualified aromatherapist. This individual will be able to choose the essential oils that will be most helpful for your condition, warn you against any potential dangers they may present, and let you know how to best apply them for maximum benefit.

Effective application of aromatherapy also begins with reliable, high-quality essential oils. These oils can be purchased from your aromatherapist, from a health food store, or through an increasing number of mail order outlets. It's important to know exactly what you are ordering as a dose of certain oils that have not been diluted enough can prove to be toxic. This is where carefully following your aromatherapist's instructions comes into play.

Additionally, the essential oils used in aromatherapy can be applied in different ways. For example, they can be inhaled, taken orally, or rubbed on the skin. Administration depends on what oil you are using, the reason you are using it, and other factors including pregnancy and asthma. This is another reason for following your aromatherapist's instructions.

The most common tool used in aromatherapy is the aroma lamp. Aroma lamps consist of a small bowl-shaped container for water, heated underneath by a small candle or light bulb. Drops of the essential oil are added to the water, with the amount depending both on the desired effect as well as the size of the room in which the lamp is being used. The heat causes the water vapor to rise into the air, along with the fragrance molecules. Lamps are generally made from glass or porcelain. Examples of oils that are helpful in allergic rhinitis reactions, and commonly used in an aroma lamp, include rose and lavender, which reduce stress, and eucalyptus or hyssop to reduce the urge to cough and to help clear up congestion.

Essential oils may also be added to a room humidifier or placed in a fragrance bowl, with water, and kept near a radiator.

A more direct means of administering aromatherapy is through inhalation. This is particularly helpful for congestion and coughs. Oil drops are added to a large bowl of steaming hot water. You then place a towel over your head, bend your face over the bowl, and breath deeply. Oils that can be used in this way include angelica and cypress to relieve sinus pain and congestion, and thyme and sage to relieve coughing. A variation of this method is to place a few drops on a handkerchief, hold it under your nose, and breathe deeply. This is especially helpful if you want to avoid the use of steam.

Aromatherapy can be administered through hot compresses. Not only does this promote relaxation, but also helps the oils penetrate deeply into the pores of the skin. To use this method, put a few drops of oil into a container of hot water. Dip a small towel into the water, wring it out, and then place it on the part of the body you want to treat. Remove the compress after it cools and, if desired, repeat this procedure with more hot water. For relaxation, use oils such as rosemary and chamomile. Ice-cold compresses can be created in the same way, using very cold water. A cold compress with mint or lemongrass can relieve the headache associated with allergic rhinitis and hay fever.

Essential oils applied directly to the skin can be useful in relieving the symptoms of allergic rhinitis and hay fever. You can easily create your own healing oils by mixing essential oils with a base oil, and then massaging this into various parts of your body. Essential oils used in aromatherapy can be easily mixed with the unprocessed or cold-processed "fatty" oils that also promote healing, such as unsaturated vegetable oils and mineral oils. Jojoba oil, wheat germ oil, olive oil, aloe vera oil, and coconut oil, all of which can be purchased at a health food store, are especially useful here.

Essential oils can be taken orally, but extreme caution is advised. Some oils can be toxic, and can lead to soft tissue irritation and negative effects on vital organs. Not only should oils be well diluted, but you should use this method only if you are working with an aromatherapist. Mint oil and lavender oil are among the oils that are safe to be taken orally; others should not be used in this way without trained guidance. Cough syrups for both adults and children, based on essential oils, can also be especially helpful.

Essential oils can also be added to bathwater or mixed with earth to create a healing poultice. These applications will be discussed in Chapter 9 (Skin Allergies and Eczema).

Botanical Medicine

Botanical medicine, also referred to as herbal medicine or herbalism, is one of the more basic healing arts and has often been referred to as the "art of simpling." Botanical medicine is relatively simple because it relies on herbs that are easy to obtain and use; it is also relatively simple because one herb can be used in treating a range of ill-

nesses, including the symptoms associated with allergic
rhinitis and hay fever.

Herbs serve three basic functions in treatment. First of
all, they promote elimination and detoxification, cleaning
the system of impurities. Herbal preparations that serve as
laxatives and diuretics assist in this process, as do those
that purify the blood. Herbs also help maintain ongoing
health by counteracting physical symptoms associated with
illness and promoting healing and recovery. Herbs also
build and strengthen the organs.

One of the main theories of herbalism is that the herbs
you need to treat your ailments are most likely available
within your geographical area. You don't always need to
travel across the country or the world to find what you
need. The reason for this local availability is that many of
your ailments, including allergies, may be related to and
even caused by the environment you live in. In the same
way that you take on the characteristics of your environment, so do herbs. Thus, the herbs that exist around you
are the ones most likely to be helpful because they build
on the healing energy of your local environment. Thus,
treating your allergies with the herbs in your environment
is somewhat similar to receiving allergy shots that contain
the allergens that most affect you.

Many herbs are relatively mild, and will have a mild
effect on your system. Thus, if you want to experience
major relief from an herb, you may want to use larger
amounts of the herb. Additionally, to experience more
dramatic and faster effects, you may need to "shock" your
system by choosing to take herbs from another environment. These herbs can be used by themselves or in combination with herbs from your geographical locale.

Herbs work in different ways, depending on the illness
you are treating and the amount of the herbs you have
chosen to treat yourself. In general, herbs should begin to

work within three days, as long as you follow the guidelines for use. These guidelines might include not only how and when to administer the herbal medication, but also associated changes you might need to make in your diet. Still, herbs are similar to the antibiotics of modern medicine in that even after the symptoms have disappeared use should be continued for a week or more to experience all of the positive effects throughout your body. When botanical medicine is applied to a longstanding, chronic condition like allergies, you may also need to continue the herbal treatment over a long period of time, even months.

How Herbs Heal In the West, herbs have traditionally been used to treat symptoms, while in other parts of the world, especially in the Orient, treatment with herbs is aimed at finding actual cures. Some practitioners in the West are expanding their view of how herbs can be used in treatment, in part because of the increased interest in natural medicines. The patients are more willing to expand their view, and thus their expectations, about what herbs can actually do.

A major reason why individuals are placing greater faith in botanical medicine is because of greater awareness of the Oriental philosophy behind the use of herbs in treating, and curing, illness. This philosophy is based on the concepts of heating and cooling energy. Each herb has its own heating or cooling energy, and subsequently each produces reactions of cooling or warmth in the body. "Warm" herbs, for example, speed the body's metabolism, while "cool" herbs slow it down. Understanding this energy, and how to use it in restoring balance to the body, is one of the keys to choosing the herbs used in treatment, and how to use them. In general, herbs with a yellow, red, or orange color produce warm energy, while those that are dark in color, including blue and purple, can be categorized as cooler herbs.

Another way to determine whether an herb is warm or cool is through its taste. Herbs with a pungent taste produce warm energy. They stimulate blood circulation and the energy of the nervous system, also stimulating the appetite and helping to reduce the production of mucus. Pungent herbs are especially useful in reducing the nasal congestion that results from allergic rhinitis and hay fever. Pungent herbs include ginger and cayenne. Salty-tasting herbs are considered sources of cool energy. They help to regulate the balance of fluids, and are useful in relaxing muscles and treating constipation. Sour-tasting herbs are also cooling, and in appropriate doses they are also useful in drying up excessive mucus production, as well as in stimulating digestion and toning muscles. Sour herbs include berries, and the peels of lemons and oranges. Bitter herbs like dandelion are also cooling, and are often used to treat inflammation. Sweet herbs can be either warming or cooling, depending on the specific herb.

Herbs are also categorized in other ways. For example, herbs move in different directions, "descending into the body," for example, or "floating on top" and drawing toxins outward. The direction of an herb depends in part on what symptoms are being treated and how the herb is being administered.

Allergic rhinitis and hay fever, as well as other allergies, can be considered either cold or warm in nature. The botanical medicine practitioner will make this diagnosis by looking closely at your overall health. Excessive mucus, for example, can be the result of a cold condition, while sore throat can be a warm condition. He or she would examine your tongue, presence or lack of sweat, and check your overall appetite and digestion, and related factors, in making a decision. In other words, botanical medicine practitioners take a broad view of allergy. Most practitioners would look closely at your individual lifestyle and eating habits, the type of symptoms you have and when, and then formulate an individual plan tailored to your needs. Herbs with specific properties would then be chosen, with the goal of reducing your symptoms and helping to fortify your body against further attacks.

The Properties of Herbs Herbs are multifaceted: one single herb can have a range of positive effects on the various organs and systems of the human body. When used in combination, these effects are multiplied. And because a single condition, like allergic rhinitis or hay fever, is associated with both a range of different symptoms as well as various debilitating effects on the body, a well-focused treatment with a variety of herbs can be useful in both treating symptoms and strengthening the body at the same time.

Herbs are generally described in terms of the effects they have on the human body. These effects are referred to as properties. Because each herb has a unique makeup that results in different reactions, depending on how it is used, a single herb may contain multiple properties.

Some of the major properties of herbs are described below, with an emphasis on those properties that are most relevant in treating allergies.

Alteratives Alterative herbs are those that are useful in altering a condition, such as arthritis, infections, skin problems, and general toxicity. Alterative herbs include echinacea, nettles, comfrey, and ginseng.

Analgesics Analgesic herbs relieve pain, including headaches associated with congestion. Herbs with analgesic properties include catnip, chamomile, and skullcap.

Antacids Antacid herbs relieve overproduction of stomach acid, like preparations you might purchase in a drugstore, while also helping to soothe and protect the stomach lining. Antacid herbs include fennel and slippery elm.

Antiasthmatics Just as the word implies, some herbs are useful in treating asthma because they help to dilate the bronchial passages and break up mucus. Antiasthmatic herbs include comfrey, coltsfoot, and mullein.

Antibiotics Herbs that help to kill germs and destroy infection, while enhancing the immune system, include chaparral, echinacea, thyme, and garlic.

Anticatarrhals Herbs with the anticatarrhal property are used to eliminate excessive mucus, generally through sweat, urine, or feces. Anticatarrhal herbs include cinnamon, anise, and sage.

Antipyretics Antipyretic herbs are those that are useful in reducing or preventing fevers, because of their ability to stimulate a cooling action in the body. These herbs include skullcap and basil.

Antiseptics Antiseptic herbs can be applied to the skin to reduce the growth of bacteria. Myrrh and garlic are examples of antiseptic herbs.

Antispasmodics Antispasmodic herbs help to relax muscle spasms so that the body can use its energy for the healing process. These herbs include valerian and rue.

Astringents   Astringent herbs are used in treating swelling and hemorrhaging, and include calendula, myrrh, and stoneroot.

Carminatives   Herbs with carminative properties are used in relieving gas and intestinal pain, and include anise, fennel, cumin, ginger, and peppermint.

Cholagogues   Cholagogue herbs act as laxatives by stimulating the elimination process, and include mandrake, wild yam, and licorice.

Demulcents   Herbs with the demulcent property are used internally to soothe inflamed tissues and to prevent tissue damage. Demulcent herbs include marshmallow, slippery elm, and chickweed.

Diaphoretics   Diaphoretic herbs are those that cause sweating, and are generally administered in the form of a very hot tea. This sweating causes toxins and other impurities to be eliminated from the system. Diaphoretic herbs include cayenne, ginger, and peppermint.

Diuretics   Diuretic herbs encourage the flow of urine, and are helpful in treating swelling, inflammation, and skin problems such as hives. Herbs that act as diuretics include horsetail, nettles, and dandelion.

Emetics   Emetics induce vomiting, allowing the stomach to empty itself of impurities that may lead to further reactions. Emetic herbs include ipecac, bayberry, and black mustard seed.

Emollients   Herbs with the emollient property are used externally to soothe and protect the skin. As such they may be especially helpful during an allergic skin reaction. Emollient herbs include comfrey root, chickweed, and marshmallow.

Expectorants   Expectorant herbs help to eliminate excess mucus through coughing. These herbs include coltsfoot, horehound, eucalyptus, and sage.

Laxatives   Laxative herbs stimulate bowel movements, and include cascara bark and rhubarb root.

Nervines   Nervine herbs promote relaxation and increased peace of mind. Depending on other symptoms and the herbs being used to treat them, a range of herbs can be used for this purpose.

Rubefacients   Rubefacient herbs are often applied to the skin, in poultices, for example, to draw congestion and inflammation out of the body. Herbs used as rubefacients include eucalyptus, cinnamon, and mustard seed oil.

Sedatives   Herbs with sedative properties have a calming effect on the nervous system similar to the nervine herbs, and include catnip, passion flower, valerian, chamomile, and skullcap.

Sialagogues   Sialagogue herbs stimulate the production of saliva, and thus aid in the process of digestion. These herbs include ginseng, cayenne, anise, dandelion, and rosemary.

Tonics   Tonic herbs have a positive and health-promoting effect on the whole body. Many herbs have this property, depending on how they are administered and which symptoms of illness are present.

The preceding list of properties is by no means exhaustive. Other herbs are used in healing wounds, inducing labor, and as aphrodisiacs.

Using Herbs in Treatment Your body will respond in a variety of ways to treatment with botanical medicine, depending on factors that include your ailment, the types and amounts of herbs used, and the way they are applied. As you will read later, ingesting herbs is not the only means of applying them. Herbs can also be used in poultices and in salves, for example.

When herbs are used in treating allergies and related conditions like anxiety, the body can have a variety of responses. One herb will eliminate toxins, and this might involve purging or sweating. Others will have a strengthening effect. It's important to keep in mind that if your allergies have placed your body in a weakened condition, using a purging herb can weaken your system even further. Thus, as with other natural treatments, it's a good idea to make sure you understand the ways in which your body might respond to an herb. Some of these responses are discussed below.

Stimulation According to botanical medicine practitioners, your body has its own natural ability to fight off illness. However, because of toxins in the environment, poor eating habits, and the stress of daily life, this ability may have been impaired. In the case of allergic rhinitis, your immune system may be so bombarded with allergens that it has at least temporarily lost the ability to discern between substances that may be harmless and those that require a defensive posture. So it has in effect turned in upon itself.

Herbs can be used to stimulate the body's natural defenses and get them back on track so that the immune system responds appropriately to the environment by ignoring the more harmless elements and standing up to those that can cause harm. Many ailments can be caused by impairments in your circulation, lymph, and other systems, resulting in areas of inactivity in your body. As a result, you may feel sluggish, and symptoms may easily manifest themselves. Herbal stimulants serve to step up your metabolism and increase your circulation. In effect, this "warms up" your body. This is especially useful when you feel an "attack" of symptoms coming on. Stimulants restore your vitality, and in essence give your system a tune-up. Herbs recognized for their usefulness as stimulants include ginger, black pepper, garlic, and cayenne.

Stimulation by herbs also helps to perk up your digestive system. The remains of foods that contribute to blockages are more quickly eliminated, including foods like sugar that in your unique makeup may cause you to be more susceptible to allergens in your environment. And if your condition also includes allergy to specific foods, the stimulating effects of herbs will also help to reduce symptoms like indigestion and cramps.

Not all stimulants are beneficial for your system, however. Some teas, for example, are acidic and can upset your stomach. Additionally, stimulants must be used carefully. For example, if your condition is a long-term one, and allergic rhinitis and hay fever certainly fit into this category, the use of stimulants can be helpful in realigning your defenses. Yet adding too much stimulation to your system, all at once, can be detrimental to an immune system that is already on "red alert" against the threat of invasion by environmental raiders. Use stimulating herbs carefully to avoid setting your system on edge. Generally, the herbal practitioner will introduce these herbs slowly, possibly in combination with other herbs that help your body to maintain its natural defenses. And if your allergy symptoms include skin problems like rashes, stimulants may serve to make this condition worse.

Tranquilization   Allergy sufferers often experience irritation and nervousness, though how your psychological states contribute to allergy symptoms is still unclear. In any case, herbal preparations that produce a calming, or tranquilizing, effect can be useful here. This not only serves to calm the immune system so that you don't react as quickly and violently to allergens, but also to create an internal environment that allows healing to go on. Calming herbs include comfrey root, and foods like barley have the same comforting effect. Other herbs, like skullcap, can be used to nourish the nervous system and bring it into balance with the other parts of your body. Tranquilizing herbs are often used in conjunction with other herbs, including those that stimulate underperforming systems, to help maintain the overall equilibrium in your body.

Blood Purification   The need to purify the blood, and thus rid it of the impurities that result from poor nutrition, environment, and lifestyle, is a major concern of botanical medicine practitioners. In fact, most practitioners view blood purification as the key to eliminating most illnesses. Your blood carries toxic substances like acids, most of which are the direct result of the chemicals we ingest and breathe. And when one of the organs of your body, or the immune system, is not functioning properly, even more toxins are added.

Herbs like dandelion can be useful in neutralizing the acids in your blood, while others stimulate organs such as the kidneys to do a better job in eliminating toxins. The herb echinacea is most often used for purifying the blood and lymphatic system.

Blood purification is usually necessary to fight infections such as pneumonia, including those that can result from an allergic reaction. Additionally, ridding the blood of toxins helps your body restore its natural defenses so that you are less susceptible to violent reactions against substances like pollen.

Tonification   Herbs can also be used to build up the energy of specific organs in your body, particularly if your energy is low and you are feeling susceptible to any illness or allergen that comes along. These herbs are referred to as tonics, and they are especially useful if you are recovering from an illness or a severe allergic reaction, as well as experiencing a chronic condition. Tonics also help you to maintain your overall good health, including the ability of your immune system to respond effectively to allergens.

Tonics provide nutrients like vitamins that nourish your organs. Some of the herbs most commonly used as tonics include seaweed and alfalfa. At any one time, some of your organs may be underperforming, while others may be working harder to compensate. This is especially true if you have had an illness or a high level of toxins in your system. Tonics help to provide balance and stimulate the energy of the organs so that the various organs of your body work more in tandem with each other.

Tonic herbs need to be used carefully. If one or more organs are underperforming, administering a tonic may increase the energy of other organs so much that the body's various organs and systems become even further out of balance. Generally, the herbal practitioner will gradually introduce milder tonics to your system, watch for the results, and then strengthen the tonics and make other adjustments as necessary.

Fluid Balance   Practitioners of botanical medicine believe that to maintain your general health, your bodily fluids must be in balance. This balance can change quickly. For example, when you experience an emotional reaction you may also experience a shift in the balance of your bodily fluids. The result might be water retention or a reduction of fluids. While many factors can affect the levels of fluids in our bodies, one factor is simply the amount of fluids we drink, either too much or too little. As with other aspects of our physical makeup, fluid balance affects our tendency toward allergic reactions, since emotional upset can make us more susceptible to the allergens around us, including pollen and mold.

Herbs such as cornsilk can help us keep the fluids in balance by acting as diuretics. Diuretic herbs stimulate the flow of urine, resulting in an elimination of toxins from the blood. Benefits can include lowering blood pressure and weight loss.

Herbal practitioners also recommend that you pay attention to your intake of fluids. If you are thirsty, your body is telling you that it needs more fluid, preferably in the form of clear, clean water. If you feel waterlogged, you may need to reduce your intake of watery foods and, especially, not drink excessive amounts of water while you are eating. This interferes with the digestive process.

Sweating Your body may respond to herbal treatment by an increase in sweating. This response is beneficial in helping to rid you of the ailments that often follow an allergic reaction, including cold symptoms and fever. Diaphoretic herbs increase the production of sweat, which then exits through your pores, taking the illness along with it and leaving you with increased strength and a feeling of well-being. Sweat-enhancing herbs include peppermint, and they are often ingested in the form of a tea.

Vomiting   Herbs that induce vomiting include syrup of ipecac, which is readily available in drugstores. Vomiting can dehydrate and weaken your system and greatly reduce your energy, thus it is not generally recommended. However, in situations where you have eaten foods that you are either allergic to or which cause you to be more susceptible to other allergens around you, vomiting may be your best and quickest defense. You should always consult your doctor for guidance on how to handle these potentially serious conditions.

Purging   Herbs can also serve as laxatives. When you are constipated, you have a buildup of toxins that can have a gradual debilitating effect on your body. As a treatment for allergy, the purging response can help cleanse your body of the toxins that render it more susceptible to pollen and other allergens in the environment. Purging is not generally recommended as an ongoing practice; like vomiting, it can leave you in a weakened state if overused. Still, herbs are preferred to the over-the-counter medicines you might purchase in a drugstore because herbs work with your body's natural responses. For example, some stimulate the production of bile, which leads to the elimination response; others serve as natural intestinal lubricants, and still others purge while also adding nutrients to your system. Work closely with your doctor and an herbal medicine practitioner when introducing purgative herbs into your system.

How Botanical Medicine Is Applied   The most common means of employing herbs is through herbal teas, depending on the specific condition being treated and the type of herbs being used. And as discussed earlier, most botanical medicine practitioners rely primarily on the herbs that are most readily available in your geographical region. Some of these herbs may be best administered by means other than through teas. Below are a few of the methods in which herbs can be used.

Herbal Teas　Many herbs that taste relatively good or at least tolerable are often administered as a tea, either hot or cold. Many herbal teas can be purchased in a health food store and may even be packaged in tea bags. However, if you choose herbs that are not in common use, you may need to visit a health food store that carries a broad line of herbs, or obtain them directly through an herbal medicine practitioner. If you purchase the herbs in bulk form, use those that have been cut and sifted so that they can easily be steeped using a tea ball.

Check for any specific instructions for brewing herbal tea. Some herbs, such as eucalyptus, require careful brewing in a tightly sealed container. Other herbs, particularly if they include plant stems, must be simmered for an hour or more. Additionally, a medicinal herbal tea often requires a large amount of the herb in order for the tea to be really effective. Generally, one ounce (25 grams) of herb is required for each pint (0.5 liter) of water, and only a couple of cups of tea may result. Thus, you will need to prepare large amounts of the tea, and save it for use at a later time. An herbal practitioner will generally direct you to drink the tea at specific periods during the day. To gain the greatest benefit, follow these directions carefully.

If possible, make your herbal tea with mineral or spring water, rather than water out of your tap, to avoid chlorine and other impurities.

Herbs may also be mixed with a sweet substance such as honey or peanut butter to make them easier to consume. This is particularly useful for herbs that have a bitter or strong taste, or when administering herbs to children.

Compress Some herbs are too strong to be taken internally. Also, the congestion associated with many forms of allergy, and asthma, responds well to treatment with herbal compresses. Hot compresses actually allow for the absorption of herbs into the body, though this is a slow process, and are a good way to administer herbs that are too strong to ingest. Herbal compresses begin with a strong herbal tea, with the cloth dipped into the tea and then applied to the area of the body being treated. The tea may be hot or cold, depending on the advice of your practitioner. Alternating hot and cold compresses may be especially beneficial in stimulating the circulation in a specific area of the body. Herbal compresses can help to break up congestion and restore vitality.

Enema Herbs like catnip are often administered in an enema, especially when being used to help reduce nervousness or to clean toxins from the blood. Enemas are generally prepared with the same amount of herb as used in herbal teas, and the solution is allowed to cool before it is administered. An enema that is too hot or too cold can irritate and even damage the bowel. Enemas should be administered carefully, under the guidance of a practitioner.

Liniment Soothing and healing herbal liniments are useful in increasing circulation as well as in treating congestion. Liniment is created by mixing herbs with vinegar, or a mixture of vegetable oils, or alcohol, and leaving it in a sealed container for a period ranging from a few days to two weeks, depending on the type of herb being used, and whether it is cut or ground. The liniment is then rubbed into the area of the body being treated. A liniment of eucalyptus herbs spread on the chest will bring warmth and increased circulation, helping to counteract the effects of allergic rhinitis and asthma.

Oils The essential oils of an herb, often used in aromatherapy treatments, are also used in botanical medicine. Herbal oils are used in a variety of ways, including internal consumption, though because of their highly concentrated nature they should be used only under the direction of a practitioner.

Poultice A poultice is a thick mass of herbs, held together by water, herbal tea, or other liquid substances and placed directly on the skin. Poultices are used to cleanse the body by drawing out toxins and infections.

Salve Herbal salves are used like liniments, though a salve is generally much thicker in consistency.

While those methods described above are the most widely used means of applying botanical medicine, there are yet others. For example, herbs may be taken in pill or gelatin capsule form. They may also be available in a syrup and, in rare instances, in herbal wine or even smoked.

While you may purchase or create your own herbal teas, or perhaps liniments or salves, botanical medicine is best used under the guidance of an experienced practitioner.

Working with a Botanical Medicine Practitioner Herbs are relatively easy to work with, and they are also safe if used externally or through packaged herbal teas. And there are a variety of excellent books on the market that can guide you in choosing and preparing your own herbal remedies. However, if you want to gain the most benefit from herbs, it is best to work with a practitioner.

As discussed previously in this section, as well as in Chapter 2, a botanical medicine practitioner, or an herbalist, will want to understand your allergy and asthma from the perspective of herbal medicine philosophy. He or she will want to know if your symptoms are the result of a hot or cold condition, and this will require understanding the general health of your body, inside and out, from your head to your extremities, the kinds of food you eat, the environment you live in, and your emotional outlook. These factors have a direct influence on how your allergies have developed and manifested themselves. The herbal treatments prescribed by your practitioner will be focused both on treating your condition as well as balancing the energies of your body.

While herbs used externally are relatively safe, take herbs internally with extreme caution, particularly if you have any food allergies. Talk with your physician before undergoing any treatment with botanical medicine to make sure that it will not interfere with other medications you may be taking.

Homeopathy

Homeopathy has an extensive history and tradition as an alternative medicine, as practiced by Dr. Samuel Hahnemann and later by Dr. Constantine Hering. Much of this history, and the basic philosophy of homeopathy, is discussed in Chapter 2. In this chapter, we'll be taking a closer look at how homeopathy can be applied in the treatment of allergy and asthma.

Homeopathy differs from many other natural treatments in that its focus is on curing the underlying illness, rather than treating the symptoms. Homeopaths believe that illness is the result of some form of stress, and as the body attempts to cope with that stress, the result is a range of symptoms. In other words, symptoms go along with illness, but they are not the actual illness.

Symptoms are manifested as the body attempts to cure itself and, even when a wide range of symptoms are present, they still represent one disease. Each medicine used in homeopathy treats one specific group of physical and psychological symptoms and it is aimed at stimulating the human body's own defenses. Thus, homeopathic medicines help the body to heal itself. In many cases, only a small stimulus—a dose of a homeopathic medicine—is needed to give the natural defenses the "jump start" necessary to complete the cycle of healing. In other cases, particularly when the illness is chronic, a longer treatment period may be required.

Because each homeopathic prescription is based on a specific group of symptoms, homeopathic physicians insist that only one medication be given at a time. This is in direct contrast to the approach of conventional medical practice in which patients are given multiple medications, sometimes one per symptom. Homeopathic physicians and manufacturers also dilute the medicines they prescribe with water or alcohol, sometimes to what seems like an extreme. This dilution is done in a specific manner, involving striking the container in a certain way and shaking it vigorously. Again, because the medicine causes symptoms that are similar to the symptoms the patient already has, homeopathic physicians believe that only a small amount is needed to promote healing.

The Homeopathic Approach to Diagnosis Homeopathic physicians take what is essentially a holistic approach to diagnosis, using a method called case taking. This is essentially an assessment of the symptoms as well as a wide range of related, and seemingly unrelated, concerns. Homeopaths ask their patients an extensive number of questions to learn about each specific symptom associated with illness, when each symptom occurs, and how it is associated with other symptoms. They also ask questions that help them in assessing a patient's mental and emotional state, looking at the presence or absence of feelings like happiness or depression, confusion or apathy, and the desire to form social relationships or to be alone. Environmental concerns and diet are also part of the case taking.

To homeopaths, symptoms are much more than just aches and pains. Symptoms include any changes that may have occurred during the course of an illness, and can include changes in attitude and emotional makeup. Case taking is generally an exhaustive and time-consuming process. If the illness is chronic in nature, like allergy and asthma, an extensive case history may also be required, including symptoms and illness experienced as a child, and immunization and medical treatment history. Homeopaths are also interested in learning more about how, in what situations, the symptoms seem to improve. For example, if your symptoms subside after drinking a cold liquid or sitting in a warm room, this information is useful in selecting the best remedy.

The Medicines of Homeopathy   The medicines used in homeopathy are derived from herbs like chamomile, comfrey, and goldenseal, as well as natural mineral sources. While they are generally nontoxic, it is still a good idea to ask about any precautions from either the practitioner or the distributor from whom you are obtaining these medicines.

Homeopathic medicines are dispensed either as drops or as pills. The dosage or potency may be increased or administered more frequently, after the initial response is assessed.

Many widely used substances, like mint or coffee, can counteract homeopathic medicines. A practitioner will caution patients as to which substances to avoid during treatment, and will also provide other dietary guidelines. While symptoms should subside rapidly after the first dose of the medicine, a few doses are generally required for healing. Severe symptoms may require repeated administrations every four hours.

If a medicine has not led to a noticeable improvement in a patient's condition after a few days, it is discontinued and another one is substituted.

Working with a Homeopathic Physician Homeopathic medicines are derived from natural sources and are relatively safe to use in treating your own allergy or asthma symptoms. And if you live in a community where no homeopathic physician is available for consultation, treating yourself in consultation with your regular doctor may be the only way to take advantage of this natural medicine option. However, it is advisable to work with an experienced and qualified practitioner, as suggested in Chapter 2. A homeopathic physician will be able to draw on his or her experience in choosing the best remedy for your specific set of symptoms, advise you as to how and when to administer it and what kinds of results to look for, and when to consider changing to another medicine.

The process of homeopathic diagnosis is discussed earlier in this section. In beginning treatment, the practitioner will first meet with you for an in-depth assessment of your condition. This will include details about each of your allergy or asthma symptoms and when they occur, to learn, for example, whether your sneezing or wheezing occurs at certain times of the day, under some circumstances and not others, and your emotional condition during these times. While you know your own symptoms much better than anyone else, and can experiment with homeopathic medicines as you desire, a practitioner can make all the difference in getting your treatment on track.

Keep in mind that homeopathic medicine is actually treating your illness with a remedy that causes similar symptoms to those that you are experiencing. Again, this is based on the philosophy of treating like with like, to restore balance to the system. If you experience a new set of symptoms, you have probably not chosen the correct remedy since, under normal circumstances for acute illness, homeopathic remedies work quickly.

Homeopathic medicine works well with improved nutrition, and your practitioner will discuss your diet with you and suggest changes. Homeopathy also works well in conjunction with meditation and exercise, as well as psychotherapy, since these approaches help to bring balance to the psyche. Avoid mixing botanical and homeopathic remedies. While both make extensive use of herbs, these preparations are used in different ways.

You should always discuss your proposed use of homeopathic remedies with your physician, especially if you are receiving treatment for your allergies on a regular basis. Many homeopathic physicians are willing and able to work with a conventional medical doctor, and some practitioners of homeopathy themselves hold medical degrees.

Naturopathy

Like other approaches to natural medicine, naturopaths view toxicity as a major cause of illness, and the connection between allergy and toxins is especially strong. Naturopaths point to a wide range of sources for toxicity. Heavy metals such as lead, nickel, and mercury are ingested into the system as a result of pollution, and they accumulate in the brain, kidneys, and the immune system. Toxic chemicals also add stress to the liver. These substances, which include alcohol, formaldehyde, and pesticides, are ingested in food, inhaled, or absorbed through the skin.

While metal and toxic chemicals can break down the body's ability to resist illness, as well as cause disorders like ulcers and chronic fatigue, it is a third kind of toxin—bacteria—that is most associated with allergic rhinitis and other forms of allergy. Bacteria and yeast, which can be consumed through food as well as inhaled, are absorbed through the gut—the digestive system—and sent throughout the rest of the body to disrupt the bodily functions. The results can include asthma and allergy, ulcers, thyroid disease, colitis, and immune disorders.

Allergies begin in the gut. To absorb our food properly, the digestive system needs to be in a balanced and relaxed, or "parasympathetic," state. However, because of a buildup of toxins in the system, the blood essentially loses its balance. The digestive system, or the gut, becomes permeable. Food particles begin to look like foreign substances to the immune system and it then reacts the same way to both toxins and harmless substances like food, and common allergens like pollen. The body forms immune complexes that are moved outward from the gut and into the extremities, where they begin to create illness.

The result is allergy, with symptoms that can take the form of allergic rhinitis and hay fever, skin allergy, food allergy, allergic reactions to air pollution, and asthma. This reaction to these "foreign substances" can also cause a variety of related illnesses. For example, the substances that the body is reacting to can lodge in the joints, and cause arthritis as the body literally eats away at its own tissues. Asthma is caused when the immune complexes lodge in the bronchial passages and cause inflammation.

Based on the belief that allergy is caused by our environment, naturopathic remedies for allergy and asthma are aimed at working with nature, instead of against it, to reach the cause of the allergy. A good analogy to think about in understanding this approach is a plant. If you place it in nutrient-rich, toxic-free soil, give it adequate light, water, and oxygen, it will thrive. Humans will also thrive in an environment with nourishment, light, clean air, minimal stress, good relationships, and a positive self-image. Because allergies result from imbalances in these elements, restoring the balance may result in a cure.

Allergy and asthma treatment may begin with the naturopath prescribing techniques to stimulate the elimination of toxin buildup, such as fasting and, in some cases, enemas. Depending on the nature of your condition, you will also be directed to avoid foods that contain certain chemicals like dyes or preservatives. Vitamin supplements may also be prescribed to correct deficiencies and build up the body's natural reserves. For allergic rhinitis, hay fever, and asthma, botanical medicines are also generally prescribed to relieve inflammation in the respiratory system. Exercise and other lifestyle modifications might also be introduced.

It's important to keep in mind that naturopaths view each individual as unique, with his or her own specific environmental conditions, lifestyle, and physical makeup. The focus of the naturopath is on correcting the internal and external imbalances that are resulting in allergy symptoms.

Working with Your Naturopath In treating patients, the naturopath has two goals. The first is to assist the patient in self-healing, and the second is to guide the patient in developing a healthier lifestyle so as to avoid further illness. During the first visit, the naturopath will learn as much about you and your illness as possible. To accomplish this, he or she will ask you detailed questions about your symptoms, your emotional condition, and your lifestyle. Of special interest will be your diet, as well as the kind of physical environment you are living in and any stress you might currently be feeling. A physical examination will be conducted, similar to the one you might receive from a medical doctor, possibly supplemented by laboratory tests and X rays.

From here, the treatment will differ among naturopaths. Some specialize in botanical medicine, and will prescribe herbal remedies, supplemented by vitamins, exercise, diet recommendations, and other traditional holistic approaches. Other naturopaths will begin with diet and other lifestyle modifications, and possibly use direct interventions like herbal medicines at a later time. The actual approach taken by the naturopath depends not only on his or her background but also on the conclusions made after examining you.

Because of the concerns that naturopaths have about the environment and its role in the development of allergy and asthma, some form of detoxification will most likely be an initial part of your treatment. Detoxification might be achieved by fasting; it is certainly the quickest way to rid the body of wastes and create a basis for beginning the healing process. A short fast generally lasts from three to five days, perhaps beginning over a weekend, and in its purest form allows only for the consumption of distilled water, though fruit or vegetable juice might be allowed. During this time, rest is recommended, as well as abstinence from any form of chemicals including soap and skin lotions. After the fast, or in place of a fast, a gradual program of detoxification is recommended. Naturopaths will often prescribe vitamin C supplements and botanical medicines to help detoxify the liver and support the lymphatic system.

Keep in close communication with your naturopath, and report both improvements as well as changes in symptoms. Also, if you are receiving regular treatment from a medical doctor, make sure that he or she is aware of your involvement in a naturopathic treatment program. Fasting, for example, is not recommended if you suffer from anemia, diabetes, or other chronic illnesses. Herbal medicines may not be compatible with other medicines you are taking. And asthma symptoms can quickly become life threatening, so it is important to have access to a medical doctor in case of an emergency.

Naturopathy is compatible with botanical medicine and homeopathy; some naturopaths draw heavily from these areas in their approach to treatment. In fact, you will most likely not need to go to a practitioner in more than one of these areas. If you do, make sure they are both aware of what you are doing. Naturopaths also make use of meditation, massage, nutrition, visualization, and other alternatives. Again, make sure your naturopath is aware of any other approaches to health that you may be practicing.

Nutrition

Chapter 2 included a discussion of nutrition and presented the basic food groups. The importance of eating a well-balanced diet, with adequate amounts of protein, fats, carbohydrates, vitamins, and minerals was emphasized. The role of fiber in the diet, along with placing a greater emphasis on fruits and vegetables, with fewer processed foods, was also discussed. You may want to review this information from time to time to make sure you are following these guidelines in your own diet.

Many of the natural approaches to treating asthma and

allergy described in this chapter, and in later chapters, also address diet. Some naturopaths, for example, specialize in nutrition, and most naturopathic practitioners will assess your diet and make recommendations. Botanical medicine practitioners, homeopathic physicians, and practitioners in areas like aromatherapy and acupressure, will most likely address nutritional issues with you. They may recommend certain foods that work well with the herbal medicines you are using, for example, but in general they will provide you with the standard guidelines for a healthy diet and encourage you to pay more attention to what you eat.

Most naturopathic practitioners believe that diet plays a role in asthma and allergies, though they differ in terms of how strong this role is, and how diet should be used in treatment. Naturopaths see a strong connection between early diet, beginning with breast-feeding, and whether or not allergies develop in later life. Other practitioners believe that certain foods can bring on allergy and asthma symptoms and, therefore, avoiding these foods can protect you from symptoms.

Nutrition experts fall somewhere in between these two viewpoints. While some allergies may be directly food related, others factors like stress, heredity, and the presence of other conditions may also be factors. And while certain foods can bring on allergy and asthma symptoms, so can airborne allergens, changes in temperature, physical exercise, air pollution, and a wide range of other factors.

Nutritionists will generally agree, however, that eating a balanced diet will help keep your body strong and fit, so that you are less vulnerable to the effects of the allergens that you normally react to. Avoiding preservatives and other additives found in food will help you to avoid loading your system with chemicals that can make you even more hypersensitive to allergens. Furthermore, some foods are associated with asthma and allergy symptoms, and these should be avoided when symptoms are present. Milk products, for example, add to mucus production and congestion, and should be avoided if you have allergic rhinitis or asthma. Eggs are associated with eczema. Additionally, depending on your own unique physical makeup, some foods may contribute to your condition while, for another person, they have no effect.

The Elimination Diet   Specific dietary recommendations for different types of allergies will be discussed where appropriate in individual chapters, especially in Chapter 10, which focuses on food allergies. Regardless of the allergy being treated, however, one of the basic tools used in determining which foods act as allergens is the elimination diet. Naturopaths use the elimination diet in discovering food allergies, and one approach to the elimination diet is discussed where appropriate in the naturopathy sections. However, the elimination diet can be approached from different perspectives.

The elimination diet, as discussed under naturopathy, is a very basic diet of a select group of foods that do not generally cause allergic reactions. This diet keeps you nourished while your body begins to detoxify itself from the chemicals and preservatives, as well as allergy-producing foods, that may be stored up. After a few days on this diet, you can begin to introduce new foods, one at a time, while watching closely for any reactions. With the elimination diet, you essentially start from the ground up in developing a diet that works for you. Once you begin to encounter foods that cause reactions, you will know which ones to avoid.

The best way to get started on an elimination diet is to work with a nutritionist who has experience in setting up such diets for individuals with allergic conditions and asthma. The nutritionist will be able to determine which foods you should start out with, how the diet should be structured, and can also give you ideas on what foods can be substituted without violating the diet. He or she will also be able to give you some recipes so that the diet doesn't get too boring. Additionally, a nutritionist can also guide you in keeping records of any reactions you experience along the way, and advise you as to when to begin introducing foods and which ones.

The specific contents of elimination diets vary among nutritionists, and are also based on your condition and your likes and dislikes. Sometimes the elimination diet is limited to a few foods, including meats, fruits, and vegetables. Your nutritionist might first recommend one diet and, if your condition doesn't improve, will then try another one.

Often elimination diets are not severe at all, at least during the early stages. For example, if your nutritionist suspects that stimulants like coffee, tea, or chocolate are contributing to your allergy symptoms, he or she might first recommend that you eliminate only stimulants from your diet, possibly for up to a month, while also eating a healthy, balanced diet. If your symptoms do indeed subside, then you can simply adopt a stimulant-free diet. If your sensitivities are more complex, you will need to go through a more rigorous elimination diet, with foods gradually introduced until you have discovered the suspected culprits.

In general, an elimination diet will include fresh, unprocessed meats and fish; potatoes, legumes, and grains; vegetables and fresh fruit; whole-grain bread; natural cereals; and to drink, spring water, unsweetened juice, and herbal tea.

Forbidden foods in an elimination diet will generally include coffee and tea; cola drinks, and any other foods or drinks that contain sugar; chocolate; liquor; any form of food coloring, preservative, food enhancer, emulsifier, or any other chemical; prepared meats like sausage; spicy food; and fast food or restaurant food. Avoiding these foods essentially eliminates the substances from your diet that are most likely to contribute to the production of histamines, and that add toxins to your system that may make you more oversensitive and more prone to allergy and asthma symptoms.

Keep in mind that you may experience a range of reactions to an elimination diet. You may feel worse because, for example, you have developed a dependency on caffeine. Or the vegetables you are eating may contain pesticide residues, or if you aren't accustomed to eating a lot of vegetables, your system may not have developed a tolerance. You may also feel better and either want to continue this diet for the long term or gradually reintroduce some of the forbidden foods, like an occasional cup of coffee, and see if symptoms begin to reappear.

A more severe elimination diet may be recommended if the one described above does not make you feel better. Other foods might need to be eliminated, such as wheat, rice, citrus fruits, yeast, peanuts, beef, or other foods that you eat on a regular basis and that you suspect may contribute to your allergy or asthma symptoms. At this point, you should work closely with your nutritionist to make sure you are meeting your basic nutritional needs. You'll need to reintroduce foods slowly, and in a certain order. Citrus fruits, for example, need to be reintroduced into your diet one at a time.

The elimination diet will also be discussed in other chapters, especially in Chapter 10, Food Allergies.

Working with Your Nutritionist We can all benefit from a healthy diet, whether or not allergy or asthma is a concern. Still, nutrition is not a miracle cure. The origins of asthma and allergy were described earlier in this chapter and what is clear is that the answers are not clear. Asthma and allergy are caused by a wide range of factors and while a better diet can help eliminate some of the factors that lead to a flare-up of symptoms, it won't eliminate all of the factors. You may feel better, but still suffer from allergy or asthma.

Work with your nutritionist on creating a diet that fits your lifestyle. Don't force yourself to eat foods you don't like when there are alternatives in the same food family. Avoid committing yourself to hours in the kitchen cooking exotic though nutritious dishes when cooking is not normally a big part of your life. And make sure your diet includes foods that are both readily available as well as affordable. To create a diet that truly meets your needs, work with your nutritionist. Be honest about your current eating habits, and what you feel most comfortable about changing, but also remain open to suggestions for changes in your diet that might really help you feel better. Follow your nutritionist's guidelines, and keep any necessary records of your intake and any symptoms you experience. The record keeping will not be fun and may even seem like a chore. It will mean recording every food item you consume, how much, and at what time of day, with any changes in how you feel. This will all be helpful as your nutritionist makes adjustments in your diet.

Avoid fad diets that promise great results, but require you to purchase expensive packaged foods. These foods may contain preservatives and empty calories and, if they become the basis of your diet, can have negative effects on your health. Whatever you need for your diet should be available in your local grocery store, health food store, and farmers' market.

Don't make radical changes in your diet without first discussing these changes with your medical doctor, especially if you are currently being treated for a specific allergic condition or asthma. Some physical conditions, like diabetes and ulcers, also may require special diet considerations. Most likely your nutritionist and your medical doctor can work together, but it's important that you communicate with both of them.

Reflexology

Reflexology is a form of massage of areas of the feet and hands called reflex points, which correspond to organs, glands, and muscles in the body. The goal of reflexology is to relieve tension through these reflex points and, at the same time, relieve symptoms of specific ailments. The basic underlying philosophy of reflexology is that the energy in your body flows through channels that terminate at the reflex points on the hands and feet. When we are feeling our best, the energy in these channels is flowing smoothly. When the energy is blocked, due to congestion or tension, illness results. Thus, by treating the reflex points, symptoms of sickness are relieved and health returns.

Generally, a reflexology session lasts less than an hour. During this time the practitioner takes one foot at a time and uses thumb and finger techniques to work with the reflex points on the sole of the foot, on the sides, and on top. Doing this correctly requires a high level of skill, since different amounts of pressure are required to get the right result. And the feet can be highly sensitive. Reflexology doesn't necessarily lead to immediate relief. Often, restoring balanced energy flow through the reflex points is a gradual process, requiring a series of sessions.

Reflexology, above all, provides a heightened sense of relaxation. But reducing your tension level can also lead to better circulation, increased nerve function, and better balance among all the various organs and systems of the body. Reflexology is also a preventive health care. By promoting relaxation and balance, it also promotes the health of the immune system, which helps in relieving the oversensitivity that can result in allergic reactions.

How Reflexology Works Like practitioners of acupuncture and shiatsu, reflexologists believe that energy flows in zones, or meridians, throughout the body. Reflexology works with ten energy zones running the length of the body from head to toe. There are five of these zones through each side of the body running from the fingertips, down through the arms, and ending in the feet. All of the organs of the body lie along one of these zones.

Each zone is a channel for life energy, called *chi*. Working with, or stimulating, a zone in the foot through reflexology techniques will affect that entire zone throughout the body. For example, working on the zone that is attached to the liver will relax and energize this organ.

Reflexologists view your foot as a miniature version of your body, with the points laid out in an arrangement similar to the organs and parts of your body. The curve of the foot is similar to the curve of your spine. Also, because the reflexology points on the foot represent all major organs of the body, this is an efficient and accessible area to use in accessing all the body parts at once. Because the feet are kept covered, they are more sensitive than the other body parts like the hands. Additionally, the feet are far away from the heart, where the blood's circulation is centered. Working with the feet brings the blood out to the extremities and increases circulation throughout the body.

Good health requires balance among all of the systems of the body. The various sources of stress in our daily lives serve to upset that balance. The condition that results is an immune system that feels attacked, and is set on edge in a fight-or-flight response. For those of us who because of other factors, like heredity, are prone to allergic reactions, our immune systems respond with oversensitivity to allergens. Sooner or later, a few granules of pollen float through the air and the sneezing begins.

Reflexology begins to treat your allergy and asthma by helping you feel as if you have entered a place of safety. This is accomplished through techniques that relax your nervous system, with special attention to the lungs, nasal passages, and the chest. Your circulation improves, and more oxygen reaches the cells, calming down the fight-or-flight tendencies of the immune system. The body is normalized and body, mind, and spirit are working as one.

Working with a Reflexologist   Reflexology is an excellent treatment for providing relaxation that can, in turn, relieve symptoms of allergy and asthma. The reflexologist will talk with you about your symptoms and overall physical condition, and will then ask you to lie on your back on a massage table and will begin working with your bare feet. This may seem strange at first, especially if your feet tend to be ticklish. Your practitioner will have his or her own style in treating you—the session may begin with the practitioner massaging the whole foot, or instead may begin by directly working with specific reflex points. Make sure you let your practitioner know when something feels good, is ticklish, or hurts. While these areas will have to be handled carefully, they may also be areas that require extra stimulation.

Unblocking the energy in your meridians may be a gradual process, and you should expect to visit your reflexologist a few times. The best way to know that reflexology is helping you is whether or not you begin to feel a greater sense of relaxation.

You can also learn a few reflexology techniques to practice on your own at home. Keep in mind, however, that reflexology requires very specific positioning of the thumb and fingers. While you can get a good idea of how this works from a book, you will be more likely to use reflexology effectively if you ask for help from your practitioner, or take a class.

Reflexology works well with meditation and breathing exercises. You may also want to have an aroma lamp in the background to help create an atmosphere of well-being and relaxation.

Reflexology can relieve some of your symptoms as a result of helping you relieve stress. It will not, however, cure your condition. You should also consult a medical doctor to be sure you are receiving the most complete treatment.

ADDITIONAL NATURAL TREATMENTS FOR ASTHMA AND ALLERGY

Additional alternatives will also be presented to you as potential treatments for asthma and specific forms of allergy. They will be introduced in the appropriate chapters. The following list includes these additional natural treatments, with a brief description of each.

Acupressure

Acupressure is an ancient art that in a sense combines acupuncture with massage. While no needles are used in acupressure treatment, it does make use of the same points as acupuncture. Acupressure practitioners believe that using the fingers to press these key points will stimulate the body's natural ability to heal itself. Like other branches of Chinese medicine, symptoms are viewed as the result of an imbalance of the energy flowing along the meridians, which connect the organs and systems of the body. Thus, allergy or asthma is viewed as the result of an imbalance that is affecting the whole body. Acupressure helps to balance the energy of the body, while also relieving tension, and increasing circulation.

While acupuncture needles can be inserted only by a qualified practitioner, you can learn to use acupressure techniques on your own to help you in relieving allergy and asthma symptoms. As long as you carefully follow the instructions, acupressure is safe to perform at home.

Affirmations

Affirmations, or self-talk, are messages that we give ourselves that define our expectations in a given situation. An affirmation can be a few words, or a sentence or more, that you say to yourself, and even write on paper, to express an outcome that you expect for yourself. You can create your own positive affirmations to help you remain relaxed and less affected by the factors that tend to set off your allergy and asthma symptoms.

Exercise

Regular physical exercise provides a multitude of benefits. It makes you look better and increases your feelings of self-esteem. It's a great release for physical and emotional tension. It builds up your stamina, including your lungs. And all of these benefits result in more empowerment, so that you don't feel like a victim of your allergies. The basic rule in setting up an exercise program is to choose an activity that fits within your own specific limitations, but that you also enjoy. Choose an activity that will get your cardiovascular system stimulated for a half hour or so, which even a brisk walk can accomplish. Don't overexert yourself, particularly when you are getting started.

Holistic Massage

Holistic massage differs from other forms of massage in that it is meditative, and focused on developing a slow, comforting relationship between the giver and the receiver. Holistic massage can be therapeutic because it promotes relaxation and feelings of well-being, provides a much-needed human connection, and helps you to become more aware of your body as a whole. Holistic massage also tones your muscles, improves your circulation, increases your hemoglobin level, and stimulates the lymph system. The result is more energy, leaving you feeling more comfortable and in control, and less reactive.

Journal Writing

In a journal you write about what you do every day, the ideas you are thinking about, how you feel about the people in your life, and what you're learning from the situations you are in. Journal writing is a way of exploring your thoughts and feelings, and working out your conflicts and fears on paper, to create a sense of relaxation and peace of mind.

Macrobiotics

The macrobiotic approach to healing is based primarily on a philosophy emphasizing the relationship of humankind with nature and the universe. Healing comes from restoring our relationship with nature, which has suffered as a result of an unnatural lifestyle and diet. Macrobiotic practitioners not only prescribe diet and lifestyle changes, but also employ a range of natural treatments, many of which are based on plants and herbs.

Meditation

Meditation is useful in relieving stress and creating inner peace and balance. This inner peace also has a calming effect on the immune system, which in turn helps to lessen the oversensitivity that can lead to allergic reaction. Most meditation techniques are based on Eastern religions where meditation is used in creating religious ecstasy. Regardless of which technique you choose to learn, it's the result—the ability to create your own state of calmness—that counts.

Psychotherapy

Psychotherapy helps you learn better ways of coping with stress, and getting what you want in life, by sorting out your past and seeing how it is still affecting you in the present. In this process, you may come to understand how your allergies and asthma fit in with your mechanisms for coping with such problems as illness and begin to see what aspects of illness you can control. You may find out you can control more than you thought. Psychotherapy can be a long and slow process, and requires a serious commitment to working through some painful and often confusing issues. If you are not ready for this commitment, there are brief forms of psychotherapy that can teach a person active coping techniques.

Shiatsu

Shiatsu is a form of massage that is useful in treating the symptoms of asthma and allergy. Shiatsu is a branch of

Oriental medicine, and is based on the concept of *chi*, the vital energy flowing along the meridians throughout the body that connect the vital organs. This same concept is used in acupressure and acupuncture, with shiatsu applying different techniques to the same points on the body. Shiatsu practitioners use their hands to detect abnormalities in the skin or muscles and make decisions as to what form of treatment to apply. Shiatsu is also holistic in nature in that it promotes the health of the entire person.

Visualization

Visualization is based on the philosophy that life is a reflection of whatever we believe, and that we rehearse these beliefs in our imagination. When you visualize, therefore, you use the power of your imagination to create mental pictures of whatever you want to experience in life. Visualization is useful both in creating a state of inner relaxation as well as promoting feelings of health and power over allergy and asthma symptoms.

Yoga

Yoga is the Sanscrit word for "reunion," which refers to the harmony between body and mind. One of the most popular yoga systems, hatha yoga, stresses the importance of body and mind awareness, and teaches various breathing and relaxation techniques to achieve this awareness. Hatha yoga techniques include deep, lung-expanding breathing, which not only helps to relax the immune system but also strengthens the lungs.

CHAPTER FOUR

Allergic Rhinitis and Hay Fever

Allergic rhinitis and hay fever are probably the most common forms of allergy, and most certainly the cause of untold hours of misery to those who suffer from them. The causes and symptoms of allergic rhinitis and hay fever in adults are discussed in this chapter, along with a range of natural treatments. Juvenile allergies are described in Chapter 5.

A DEFINITION OF ALLERGIC RHINITIS AND HAY FEVER

The terms "allergic rhinitis" and "hay fever" are often used interchangeably, but there is a subtle difference between the two conditions. Hay fever is caused by the pollen of certain flowers. Not all pollens cause hay fever, however; generally it is the light, airborne pollens of trees, grasses, and weeds, which are present in the spring, as well as the pollen from ragweed, which appears in the late summer. As a result of this pattern, hay fever tends to be a seasonal condition, tormenting allergy sufferers during the spring and fall.

Allergic rhinitis differs from hay fever primarily because those who have this condition can suffer during all four seasons. While allergic rhinitis sufferers are sensitive to pollen, mold, and other substances produced by nature, they may also be sensitive to allergens like smoke, perfumes, window cleaners, industrial pollution, insect repellants, plant-care products . . . the list is almost endless. What these allergens have in common is that they are inhaled.

Allergic rhinitis and hay fever are also similar to each other in terms of the kind of symptoms they produce. Allergic rhinitis symptoms include nasal stuffiness, sneezing, sniffing, runny nose, postnasal drip, and often, an impaired ability to smell. Most people with allergic rhinitis find that symptoms are more severe in the morning, and while outdoors. Hay fever symptoms are similar. They include runny or itchy eyes and nose, sneezing, red and swollen eyes, itchy soft palate and ears, and sometimes a rash.

The Main Culprit: Pollen

One thing that most allergic rhinitis and hay fever sufferers have in common is an allergy to pollen. In fact, most allergies involving the nose, eyes, and lungs are caused by plant pollens. Plants produce microscopic round or oval pollen grains in order to reproduce. In some species, the plant uses the pollen from its own flowers to fertilize itself. Other types must be cross-pollinated, or transferred from the flower of one plant to the flower of another plant of the same species. This task might be carried out by insects or by wind transport.

The pollens most likely to cause allergic reaction are produced by certain weeds, trees, and grasses lacking conspicuous flowers. The pollens produced by these plants are small, light, dry, and easily transported granules. Ragweed samples have been collected four hundred miles out at sea and two miles high in the air. Also, these plants may produce huge quantities of pollen, millions of grains of pollen a day from one plant.

The chemical makeup of pollen is the basic factor that determines whether it is likely to cause hay fever. A heavy pollen, like pine pollen, falls straight down to the ground and is less likely to be inhaled by humans. Conspicuous wildflowers or the flowers in most gardens also generally produce a heavy pollen less apt to be inhaled by humans. Lighter pollens, like ragweed, are much more likely to be airborne. Other allergy-causing pollens include sagebrush, redroot pigweed, lamb's quarters, Russian thistle (tumbleweed), and English plaintain. Grasses that produce allergic pollen include timothy, Johnson, Bermuda, redtop, orchard, sweet vernal, and Kentucky bluegrass. Trees that produce allergic pollen include oak, ash, elm, hickory, pecan, maple, and mountain cedar.

It is difficult to escape pollen because the particles can be carried significant distances. Thus, it is important for you not only to understand local environmental conditions but also conditions over the broader area of the state or region in which you live and work.

Geographical Cures: Pollens by Region and Season Because pollen is seasonal, hay fever sufferers will experience reactions only at certain times of the year. Each plant has a pollinating season that is more or less the same every year, depending on the geographical location. The pollen count—the amount of pollen in the air—is expressed in grains of pollen per cubic meter of air collected over twenty-four hours. Pollen counts are highest early in the morning on warm, dry, breezy days. Counts are lowest during chilly and wet days.

Here is a list of major pollens, organized by region of the United States, and by season. This information was compiled by the Asthma and Allergy Foundation of America.

NORTHEAST

Tree Pollens

March–May   birch (especially in New England), oak,
                     sycamore, elm, maple, ash, poplar,
                     beech, hickory, walnut

*Grass
Pollens*

May–July   orchard grass, bluegrass, timothy, redtop

Weed Pollens

August–   ragweed, Russian thistle, hemp, red
September   sorrel, plantains, pigweed, Mexican
                     firebrush

SOUTH AND SOUTHEAST

Tree Pollens

February–   red cedar, mulberry, pecan, elm, maple,
June   poplar, ash, oak, birch, alder, beech,
                     sycamore, hickory, walnut, elm, pecan,
                     bayberry, cypress

*Grass
Pollens*

June–
September   Bermuda, timothy, natal

Weed Pollens

August–
September   ragweed

MIDWEST

Tree Pollens

March–May   elm, maple, poplar, ash, oak, birch,
                     alder, sycamore, walnut, hickory

*Grass
Pollens*

May–July   orchard grass, bluegrass, timothy

Weed Pollens

| August–
September | ragweed, Russian thistle, hemp,
pigweed, lamb's quarters, red sorrel |

SOUTH CENTRAL

Tree Pollens

| January–April | oak, hackberry, elm, mountain cedar,
pecan, red cedar |

*Grass
Pollens*

| May–July | Bermuda, Johnson |

Weed Pollens

| August–
October | ragweed, Russian thistle |

SOUTHWEST

Tree Pollens

| March–May | mountain cedar, Chinese elm,
cottonwood, ash, sycamore, walnut |

*Grass
Pollens*

| April–
October | Bermuda grass, bluegrass, brome,
redtop, orchard, barn rye |

Weed Pollens

| April/June–
September | tumbleweed, firebrush, ragweed, sage |

NORTHWEST

Tree Pollens

| March–May | alder, birch, oak, maple, hazel, walnut,
sycamore, elm, cottonwood, birch, ash,
fruit trees |

*Grass
Pollens*

| May–July | bluegrass, timothy, orchard, rye, brome,
oat, redtop, velvet |

Weed Pollens

August–September	tumbleweed, sagebrush, Russian thistle, ragweed, amaranth

WEST

Tree Pollens

March–May	elm, maple, oak, ash, alder, sycamore, hickory, walnut, poplar

Grass Pollens

March–May	bluegrass, timothy, orchard

Weed Pollens

March–May	sagebrush, ragweed, tumbleweed

Will moving to one of these regions help you to avoid allergic reactions? Practitioners do not generally recommend that their patients move to a new geographical location to avoid allergens. No area of the country is truly allergen free. You may avoid a particular pollen in one location only to discover a new grass allergy in another. And with shifting winds, inhalants can be blown into other areas anyway. You may want to consider taking a vacation during your worst allergy weeks and escape to a desert or a beach.

Mold Allergy

Molds are a major cause of allergic rhinitis during certain seasons of the year, generally from spring to late fall, with a peak from July to late summer. Molds are actually plants in the fungus family. The seeds of fungi are called spores, each species producing spores that differ in size, shape, and color. Each spore that germinates results in the growth of new molds, and each of these molds can in turn produce millions of spores. While there are thousands of different types of molds, fortunately, only a few types actually cause allergy.

Mold spores can cause allergic rhinitis when they are inhaled. Because they are microscopic in size, they easily get past the protective mechanisms of the nose and upper respiratory tract. As a result, they can also cause asthma symptoms with a buildup of mucus, wheezing, and difficulty in breathing.

Molds grow wherever there is moisture, oxygen, and a source of the other chemicals they need to flourish. They are especially prevalent in the fall, when they grow on rotting logs and fallen leaves. Molds are also found in the compost piles of gardens, and can attach themselves to grains like wheat and barley. Inside of the home, molds flourish in damp basements and closets, as well as in bathrooms. They also grow on house plants, in humidifiers, air-conditioners, and garbage pails. Like pollen, molds are light enough to be carried by air currents. In some cases, they may even be more prevalent in the air than pollen.

Molds are also much more persistent than pollen. While pollen generally disappears after the first frost of the fall, molds may persist because some can grow at sub-freezing temperatures. While snow can lower the amount of mold found outdoors, it does not kill it. And after spring thaw, molds thrive on the vegetation that has been killed by the winter cold. In areas of the country that stay warm through the year, mold can cause year-round allergy symptoms.

Individuals with severe mold allergy can also experience symptoms as a result of eating certain foods like cheese, which contain fungi. Mushrooms and dried fruits, as well as foods containing yeast, like soy sauce, can also cause an allergic reaction.

Dust Allergy

The most common cause of year-round allergic rhinitis is house dust. Regardless of how clean your house is, dust manages to find its way inside. And if you have a sensitivity to house dust, your allergies may be as severe in the winter as during the other seasons, with forced-air heating systems blowing dust particles into your air.

House dust is really a generic term. Instead of being a single substance, house dust is made up of a wide range of materials, including the fibers from different types of fabrics like cotton lint, and feathers or down, as well as bacteria and human skin particles. It may also contain mold and fungus spores, parts of plants, and food particles.

House dust also contains mites, which are microscopic creatures that live in upholstered furniture, carpets, and bedding. Mites can thrive throughout the winter if your house is warm and humid. These mites and their waste products, as well as cockroaches and their waste products, can set your allergic rhinitis on edge.

House dust, because it is made up of so many different substances, varies greatly from one home to another. And while good housekeeping can help keep house dust to a minimum, even the tiniest amount can cause allergic reactions in people with house-dust sensitivities. Furthermore, as far as dust mites are concerned, no amount of vacuuming and dusting will reduce the numbers of mites that have burrowed deep within your carpets.

Animal Allergy

Does Fido make you sneeze? Household pets, as lovable and affectionate as they seem, can cause violent allergic reactions in people with animal allergies. Animal fur was long thought to be the cause of allergic reactions to animals. It is now believed that it is the animal saliva that causes allergic reactions. Animals lick themselves when they preen, depositing this saliva in their fur. Once this saliva dries, it becomes airborne along with the fur and is thus inhaled by allergic humans. Cats are the pet most likely to cause reactions because they preen themselves more than other animals, and they spend more time in the house. Other furry pets like guinea pigs and gerbils can also cause allergic reactions as a result both of their saliva and urine.

If you recently acquired a household pet and haven't yet experienced an allergic reaction, you're not yet in the clear. It can take as long as two years for an animal allergy to develop. And the allergens they give off can get into your furniture and carpet, remaining active for months. So if you decide to find another home for your pet, it may take a few months before your house is free of pet-related allergens.

FACTORS THAT CAUSE ALLERGIC RHINITIS AND HAY FEVER

No one really knows exactly what causes allergic rhinitis and hay fever. As with other forms of allergy, the causes are varied and complicated. Some of these factors are discussed below.

Heredity

Allergic rhinitis and hay fever are often inherited conditions. The tendency to be allergic to specific substances—mold, for example, as opposed to cat hair—may be inherited as well. You may be able to pinpoint the parent, or close relative, who most likely passed their allergies on to you. Heredity is only one factor in the development of allergies; it is also possible that you are the only member of your family who can't be around a dog without sneezing.

The Environment

Over the last few decades, our environment has become increasingly polluted. Inhaling industrial waste and other chemicals, as well as tobacco smoke, can cause long-term damage to the respiratory system, including increased susceptibility to allergic rhinitis and hay fever. If you already have a genetic predisposition, chances are environmental conditions can make the situation worse.

Food Additives

There is a strong connection between diet and allergy. Consuming a diet heavy in food additives adds toxins to the system that can make you even more susceptible to allergic rhinitis and hay fever.

Emotions

Strong negative emotions, like anger, frustration, and stress, can weaken your immune system, making it more likely that a condition like allergic rhinitis will develop, especially if you have a genetic predisposition.

While you can't do much about your genes, and exposure to the environment and food additives may already have played a role in the development of your allergies, you can still do something about this condition. And the first action to take is avoiding the allergens that cause your allergic rhinitis symptoms. Avoidance begins at home.

Where to Start: Making Your Home Allergy Free

You've heard the old cliché "Charity begins in the home." So does treatment for your allergies. If your home is dirty, dusty, and full of the allergens that cause your allergic rhinitis to flare up, you're going to be short-circuiting your own health. You can supplement any treatment you choose by making your environment at home as allergy free as possible. Here is a list of some of the steps you can take.

- Avoid carpeting—it hides house dust and animal dander. Bare wood and tile floors are much easier to keep clean.

- Use only washable window shades and curtains. Venetian blinds and heavy drapes are places for dust to hide.

- Use polyester or foam pillows instead of feather pillows.

- Keep the bedroom free of dust-catching furniture and bookshelves, as well as stuffed animals.

- Change the furnace and air-conditioning filters often to avoid recirculating dust.

- Use easily washable blankets, and wash them often. Down comforters and quilts can hold dust and leak tiny allergenic feathers.

- Eliminate all smoking from the house.

- Enclose mattresses and pillows in allergy-proof encasings, to protect from dust, mites, and mold.

- Make sure your dryer is vented to the outside of the house, so that dust and molds are not vented inside.

Surface dust can keep your allergies on edge throughout the year, but you can help control your own allergy risks by keeping dust to a minimum. Vacuum often, and dust with a damp or oiled cloth. When you dust, wear a dust mask or, if possible, ask a nonallergic person to do your dusting for you. Also remove dust-collecting items from your house. For example, upholstered furniture collects and holds dust, while leather and wood furniture does not. Buy bookcases and cabinets with doors rather than using open shelves where dust can collect.

Because allergies are often worse at night, as is asthma, the bedroom deserves special attention. Follow the above guidelines in ridding your bedroom of dust and other allergens. In addition to using foam pillows and avoiding dust-collecting comforters and bedspreads, also keep your closet door closed. Dust can collect on the clothes and other items stored there, and this dust can end up floating through the air you breathe while you sleep.

You can also control your environment at home. Use air conditioning to keep the inside air free of the humidity that encourages mold and mite growth. If you don't have an air-conditioner in the bedroom, consider adding one. Also clean the air-conditioner filter often and replace the furnace filters.

And after you have finished with preventive measures like cleaning your house, you can move on to exploring ways of treating your symptoms.

TREATING YOUR ALLERGIC RHINITIS AND HAY FEVER WITH NATURAL MEDICINE

As with other allergies, the natural medicine approach to allergic rhinitis and hay fever is holistic rather than specific. For example, a medical doctor will test you for allergy to specific substances, like certain types of pollen, mold, and animal saliva. Your treatment will then probably include allergy shots to desensitize you to these specific allergens, supplemented by decongestants and antihistamines to relieve your symptoms. Natural medicine, on the other hand, takes a broader approach.

Most practitioners recognize the role of heredity in allergic rhinitis and hay fever, and view symptoms as having their roots in the immune system. However, rather than focusing on specific allergens and how they affect you, natural medicine treatment will be oriented toward the connection among your mind, body, and spirit. This might include healing the imbalances in your system that are causing overreactions to inhaled allergens, through treatments such as acupuncture and botanical medicine. Treatment might also include relieving the stress that makes your immune system vulnerable, through practices such as meditation and visualization. Natural medicine alternatives will also include recommendations on improving your outlook on life, and making changes in your lifestyle, especially regarding diet and exercise.

Natural medicine offers a range of options for treating your allergic rhinitis and allergy. Many of these options are described in this chapter. However, don't make decisions about treatment without talking to your physician. And before you decide to discontinue any allergy medications, discuss the potential implications of this decision with your physician, as well as with your practitioner.

NATURAL TREATMENTS FOR ALLERGIC RHINITIS AND HAY FEVER

Acupuncture

Acupuncture, discussed in Chapter 3, can control as well as eliminate your allergic rhinitis and hay fever symptoms. Receiving acupuncture treatments from a qualified practitioner, during the season before your symptoms actually occur, can be especially helpful. For example, treatments during the winter months can bolster your system before the onslaught of spring pollen.

Acupressure

Acupressure is a form of massage, based on the same philosophy, and using the same points of the body, as acupuncture. Acupressure employs very specific techniques in applying pressure to stimulate the body's natural ability to heal itself. This stimulation causes endorphins to be released, which are chemicals that relieve pain and reduce stress. This helps the body to regain its internal balance and enhances the ability of the immune system to work effectively.

Like acupuncturists, acupressure practitioners view symptoms as the result of an imbalance of the energy flowing along the meridians, which connect the organs and systems of the body. Allergic rhinitis is viewed as the result of an imbalance that is affecting the whole body. Acupressure helps to rebalance the energy of the body, while also relieving tension, and increasing circulation.

Symptomatic acupressure treatment can relieve the congestion and sneezing associated with allergic rhinitis and hay fever. Specific acupressure points on the body can be used to relieve these symptoms by redirecting the flow of energy and promoting healing. While this type of acupressure does not offer a cure as such, it can be used to reduce symptoms before they become severe. With practice, acupressure can even be used to help prevent allergy symptoms. To help resolve the underlying energetic imbalance, it would be more effective to get regular acupuncture treatments.

Acupressure Guidelines

When practicing acupressure on your own, following a few basic guidelines will help to assure that you benefit as much as possible. First of all, always wear comfortable, loose-fitting clothing. And sit, or lie down, depending on the treatment, in a quiet room where you won't be disturbed. Soft music can also help to create a calming atmosphere.

The acupressure points are at the surface of the skin, so you don't have to press so hard that you bruise yourself. Some techniques may require that the acupressure point be pressed firmly. However, generally a light touch is all that is necessary. What is most important is that you carefully follow instructions to find the exact location of the acupressure point. Most acupressure points are located in slight indentations under the skin. When you locate it, you may feel a bit of soreness or a tingling sensation. As you develop your own skills in applying acupressure, keep your focus on finding the acupressure points and lightly stimulating them. As you become more proficient, and your technique matures, stimulating the proper point will become second nature.

Relieving Your Allergic Rhinitis Symptoms with Acupressure   Below are some exercises that can help relieve your allergic rhinitis and hay fever symptoms. Try them on your own or ask a friend to help you.

Sneezing and Nasal Congestion   Relief from sneezing, nasal congestion, and sinus pain begins with the hand. One of the body's antihistamine points, in Chinese medicine called Joining the Valley, is located in the center of the webbing between the thumb and index finger (the large intestine, point number LI 4 on the chart). Locate this point and gently apply pressure by placing your right thumb on top of the center of the webbing of your left hand. Gently press on it with the right thumb, angling the pressure toward the bone that connects with your left index finger. Take deep steady breaths while continuing to press. This should be continued for up to one minute. Repeat the exercise on the other hand.

Also use your index fingers to press between the bones on the top of your feet at the point that lies between the large toe and the second toe (the liver, at point number Lv 3). Rub this area firmly, angling the pressure toward the bone that connects with the second toe.

Headache and Swollen Eyes   Symptoms like headache and swollen eyes can be relieved by applying pressure at the point that lies one half inch below the base of the skull, called the Heavenly Pillar (B 10). This area is located on the muscles on either side of the spine. Use your thumbs and press firmly on both sides for one minute.

Watery Eyes and Head Congestion   To gain relief for watery eyes and head congestion, begin by pressing the bridge of the nose between your thumb and index finger. Press upward into the indentations of the eye sockets. With the other hand, use your fingertips to grasp both sides of the back of your neck. Use your fingertips on the left side and the heel of your hand on the right side to firmly squeeze the neck muscles. Close your eyes and hold these points for at least one minute as you breathe deeply.

Working with an Acupressure Practitioner Acupressure can lead to relief from your allergy symptoms. However, it is not magic. Making it work for you requires that you carefully follow the directions of the practitioner and perform the exercises as directed. If your allergy symptoms do not subside, or if others develop, you should report this to the practitioner so that your treatment routine can be readjusted. If positive change does not occur, the treatment may not work for your condition. Acupressure is a good complement to herbal remedies and meditation.

Affirmations

Most likely, when you come into contact with an allergen, or feel an allergic reaction coming in, you start telling your body to get ready for the attack. For example, when you hear the weather report on the radio, and the announcer mentions a high pollen count, you say something to yourself like "I'll be sneezing my way through this day." Even if you aren't necessarily conscious of these messages, chances are you're expecting the worse.

Affirmations, or self-talk, are messages that we give ourselves that define our expectations in a given situation. Self-talk can be positive or negative, depending on what you expect. When your allergies are bothering you, you can use positive self-talk, with affirmations that remind you that you do not have to be a victim of pollen or cat hair or whatever other substance is threatening you. In fact, by using affirmations, you are redefining an allergen as a neutral, harmless substance that you don't have to have a reaction to. Practicing affirmations can help you to maintain a positive focus on getting better and, when in the midst of an allergic reaction, produce a calming affect that can in turn calm the immune system and reduce symptoms. Here are a few affirmations to use for allergic rhinitis and hay fever:

- Cat hair is just cat hair. It's not a threat to me.
- I love springtime and nature's constant renewing of itself. I enjoy the trees and flowers.
- My allergy symptoms are disappearing. I don't need to be allergic.
- The world is a safe and friendly place. I feel protected.

Choose the allergens that you are most sensitive to and create affirmations that counteract their effects on you. Write the affirmations on paper or on small cards and keep them handy as reminders of positive self-talk. You may even want to tape them up over your kitchen sink or near the bathroom mirror to keep yourself focused.

The best time to say affirmations is during the morning, when your mind is fresh, as well as in the evening before bedtime. You may also want to record your affirmations on tape and then play it when you're driving or working around the house.

A wide range of books are available that describe the use of affirmations and teach you how to write your own.

Aromatherapy

Here is the key to how aromatherapy can help you with allergy relief: While you can breathe in allergens that result in allergic rhinitis and hay fever reactions, you can also breathe in relief by using aromatherapy techniques.

Aromatherapy can be administered through hot compresses. Not only does this promote relaxation, but also helps the oils penetrate deeply into the pores of the skin. To use this method, put a few drops of oil into a container of hot water. Dip a small towel into the water, wring it out, and then place it on the part of the body you want to treat. Remove the compress after it cools and, if desired, repeat this procedure with more hot water. A cold compress with mint or lemongrass can relieve the headache associated with allergic rhinitis and hay fever. Essential oils applied directly to the skin can be useful in relieving the symptoms of allergic rhinitis and hay fever.

The following are essential oils that can be helpful in treating the symptoms of allergic rhinitis and hay fever. Alternatives for using these oils in applying aromatherapy are suggested.

Angelica   Angelica is a tall plant common in temperate regions. The essential oil is taken from its roots. To treat congestion and breathing problems, use two or three drops of angelica in an aroma lamp three times per day. When used in a massage oil, angelica also improves circulation and promotes general health.

Balm   The balm plant is a member of the mint family, and is grown throughout the world, including North America. It has a long history of use in treating anxiety, depression, irregular heartbeat, and breathing problems. Balm is also used by aromatherapists in treating allergic rhinitis and hay fever, helping to reduce symptoms through its healing properties. To use balm for allergy relief, add a few drops to an aroma lamp. Two or three drops can also be taken orally.

Cedar   Cedar oil is extracted from the bark of the cedar tree, grown mainly in Morocco. The use of cedar goes back to the early Egyptians who used it as an insect repellant and for mummification, and through the centuries its healing properties also became apparent. Cedar is helpful in treating bronchial ailments and the cough associated with allergic rhinitis, helping to clear the passages and also acting as an expectorant. It can be taken orally, with up to two drops added to water, twice daily. A few drops of cedar can also be added to an aroma lamp.

Immortelle   Immortelle is a flowering plant that grows in tropical America. Its oil is recognized as a treatment for chronic ailments, particularly those that relate to the skin, lymph system, and mucous membranes. As such it is beneficial for allergy sufferers, as well as those affected by environmental and industrial irritants. For treating allergic rhinitis and hay fever, a few drops of immortelle should be mixed with water in an aroma lamp. Immortelle also works well in combination with angelica.

Depending on your specific allergies, some essential oils will work better with others. Try a few different oils, alone and in combination, and discover which ones work best for you. If you do not notice any improvement from inhaling these oils, and especially if you feel the oils may be contributing to your allergies, you should discontinue this treatment.

Botanical Medicine

Many of your ailments, including allergies, are related to and even caused by the environment you live in. In the same way that you take on the characteristics of your environment, so do herbs. Thus, the herbs that exist around you are the ones most likely to be helpful because they build on the healing energy of your local environment. Thus, treating your allergies with the herbs in your environment is somewhat similar to receiving allergy shots that contain the allergens that most affect you.

Allergic rhinitis and hay fever, as well as other allergies, can be considered either cold or warm in nature. The botanical medicine practitioner will make this diagnosis by looking closely at your overall condition. Excessive mucus, for example, can be the result of a cold condition, while sore throat can be a warm condition. He or she would evaluate the condition of your tongue, presence or lack of sweat, and check your overall appetite and digestion, and related factors, in making a decision. Herbs with specific properties would then be chosen, with the goal of reducing your symptoms and helping to fortify your body against further attacks.

Herbs are multifaceted: one single herb can have a range of positive effects on the various organs and systems of the human body. When used in combination, these effects are multiplied. And because a single condition, like allergic rhinitis or hay fever, is associated with both a range of different symptoms as well as various debilitating effects on the body, a well-focused treatment with a variety of herbs can be useful in both treating symptoms and strengthening the body at the same time.

When herbs are used in treating allergies and related conditions like anxiety, the body can have a variety of responses. One herb will eliminate toxins, and this might involve purging or sweating; others will have a strengthening effect. It's important to keep in mind that if your allergies have placed your body in a weakened condition, using a purging herb can weaken your system even further. Thus, as with other natural treatments, it's a good idea to make sure you understand the ways in which your body might respond to an herb.

The following are examples of herbs that are often used by botanical medicine practitioners in treating allergic rhinitis and hay fever. You should not undertake any herbal therapy, however, without first consulting with your doctor.

Astralagus   Astralagus, a sweet-tasting root, is used in strengthening and energizing the body, and in treating illnesses such as colds and flu. It is particularly effective in treating lung problems and is thus useful in treating the symptoms of allergy, particularly lung congestion and weakness. Astralagus can be cooked in soups, or with grains, as well as used in tea.

Damiana   The leaves of the damiana plant, a spicy-tasting herb, are useful in treating the congestion that can accompany an allergic reaction. To use damiana in an herbal tea, follow these directions:

1. Place one ounce of damiana herb in a teapot.
2. Boil one pint of water in a separate container and then pour it into the teapot containing the damiana.
3. Cover the teapot and let it steep for at least fifteen minutes.
4. Strain the herb fragments out of the tea and drink it warm or cool.

Ginko   Ginko is taken from the nuts and leaves of the ginko tree, is bitter tasting, and can be mildly toxic. Ginko is highly useful as an expectorant; it expels mucus from the lungs, as well as relieving the coughing and wheezing associated with both asthma and allergy. Ginko can be purchased in the form of an extract, but also taken in a tea. Because of its potentially toxic nature, particularly when ginko nuts are used, it is best used under the guidance of a botanical medicine practitioner.

Mustard   The use of mustard seed has a long history as a folk remedy. It is useful in stimulating circulation and relieving congestion. When used in treating allergies, mustard can be administered in the form of a plaster that is placed on the chest. To make one, mix one tablespoon of mustard powder with four tablespoons of flour, preferably whole wheat, and make a thick paste by adding a little water. Spread this mixture on a cotton cloth, and lay it on your chest. You may want to first lay a plain piece of cloth on your chest as protection from direct contact with the mustard. Remove it after you start to experience a burning sensation.

Peppermint   Peppermint has long been used as a medicinal herb and it is useful in treating a variety of conditions, including nasal and chest congestion. To make an herbal tea, use one ounce of peppermint herb and follow the above directions. A few drops of peppermint oil can also be dropped into the boiling water, and the contents inhaled to open nasal passages.

Herbs are relatively easy to work with, and they are also safe if used externally or through packaged herbal teas. And there are a variety of excellent books on the market that can guide you in choosing and preparing your own herbal preparations. However, if you want to gain the most benefit from herbs, it is best to work with a practitioner.

As discussed previously in this section, as well as in Chapter 2, a botanical medicine practitioner or an herbalist will want to understand your allergies from the perspective of herbal medicine philosophy. He or she will want to know if your symptoms are the result of a hot or cold condition, and this will require understanding the general condition of your body, inside and out, from your head to your extremities, the kinds of food you eat, the environment you live in, and your emotional outlook. These factors have a direct influence on how your allergies have developed and manifest themselves. The herbal treatments prescribed by your practitioner will be focused both on treating your condition as well as balancing the energies of your body.

While herbs used externally, under the guidance of a practitioner, are generally considered safe, take herbs internally (other than packaged teas) with extreme caution, particularly if you have any food allergies. Talk with your physician before undergoing any treatment with botanical medicine to make sure that it will not interfere with other medications you may be taking.

Holistic Massage

The hypersensitivity associated with allergic rhinitis and hay fever can in part be a result of feelings like anxiety, anger, loneliness. When these feelings sit around in our system, they keep us on edge, and when they are finally expressed, they may come out in symptoms like sneezing and coughing. Holistic massage is not a cure for these feelings, but it can be useful in promoting relaxation and feelings of well-being.

Giving a Holistic Massage The individual receiving the massage is generally nude, or at least minimally clothed. The session begins with the receiver lying on his or her stomach, on a comfortable mat on the floor, while the giver gently applies oil. Coconut or vegetable oil can be used for this purpose. Also, properly diluted essential oils can add an additional therapeutic dimension to this process, particularly jasmine and tangerine oil. Touch is at first very gentle, caressing the back with the oil and gradually moving toward the part of the body that is going to be massaged first.

There are literally hundreds of strokes you can use in holistic massage. Some of the basics include long, gliding strokes, moving the surface of the hands up and down along the curves of the body. Another stroke, called feathering, involves lightly touching the skin with the fingertips, alternating hands, to promote relaxation. Strokes that involve applying more pressure include a kneading motion in which the giver grasps and squeezes an area of flesh, alternating hands in a rhythmical motion. Strokes that are particularly beneficial in stimulating circulation include using the side or heel of the fists to pummel the flesh lightly, again with one fist after the other in rhythm. The sequence of holistic massage begins with the back, moving to the back of the legs, to the shoulders, neck and scalp, to the face, the hands and arms, and then on to the front of the torso and legs.

Allergic rhinitis and hay fever sufferers often carry tension in their chest and shoulders as a result of constant sneezing and chest congestion. Pay close attention to these areas by spending more time massaging the upper back, as well as the chest and shoulder areas. This includes kneading the pectorals and using the fingers to press between the ribs. Promoting relaxation and balance in these areas can help to relieve hypersensitivity.

As mentioned earlier, the essential oils of aromatherapy can be diluted to use as massage oils, and using an aroma lamp during a massage session can help to create a relaxing environment. Massage is universally compatible with other natural approaches to treating allergic rhinitis and hay fever and, unless you or the person you are massaging has a physical condition that prevents being touched, like a skin inflammation, it presents few risks.

Homeopathy

The goal of homeopathy is to help the natural healing process along so that the cycle of stress-illness-symptoms is broken. The homeopathic view of allergy is consistent with this approach. The symptoms of allergic rhinitis—sneezing, coughing, and runny eyes, for example—indicate a troubled immune system.

When the immune system is working at its peak, it is able to distinguish the more innocuous germs and substances from those that might result in conditions like cancer. Homeopaths would agree with other practitioners that, in the case of allergic reaction, the immune system is also defending itself against normally harmless substances like pollen. As further evidence of an underlying cause, symptoms may also develop as a response to changes in temperature, after exercise, and in response to emotional upset. Homeopaths view allergic rhinitis and other allergies as oversensitivity. Like practitioners of conventional medicine, homeopaths are not able to pinpoint exactly why this imbalance leads to allergic rhinitis, as opposed to other allergies, or other ailments altogether. The homeopathic approach to allergic rhinitis and hay fever is aimed at correcting the internal imbalances that result in the allergic symptoms.

If you are being treated by a physician, you are most likely receiving antihistamines and decongestants to help you gain the upper hand over sneezing and congestion. Homeopaths take a dim view of these drugs because they merely mask the symptoms of the internal imbalance, and they suppress the body's own natural defenses. Furthermore, if you continue using these drugs indefinitely, your body can develop a tolerance that renders the drugs less effective. And according to homeopaths, if the imbalance continues to go untreated, while the symptoms are being suppressed, your body produces other and possibly more dramatic symptoms.

Conventional medicine also treats allergic rhinitis and hay fever through immunization, with specific allergens injected on a regular basis to desensitize or "wear out" the allergy. Based on the homeopathic philosophy of treating illness with substances that in effect mimic the current symptoms, this makes sense. However, many homeopathic practitioners question the use of desensitization injections. Allergy shots contain specific allergens that are known triggers. Individuals can be allergic to a range of allergens that go beyond those that are contained in the injection so, again, the underlying imbalance may be modified but not cured. Additionally, the allergens being used may lead to further allergic reactions rather than lead to tolerance.

While the aim of homeopathic medicine is to cure underlying imbalances, diagnosis is based on the specific symptoms that are being exhibited. This is not to imply that a homeopathic physician will advise you to take a range of medicines, one for each symptom. Instead, he or she will treat you with one specific homeopathic medicine at a time. The medicine chosen is closely matched with the group of symptoms that you are exhibiting.

Below are the major homeopathic medicines used in treating allergic rhinitis and hay fever, with the associated symptoms. Generally, these medicines should be obtained from a qualified practitioner, and used under his or her guidance. However, because these preparations are based on herbs and other natural substances, you can also obtain and safely use them on your own, after checking first with your treating physician. Instructions for using these remedies are provided later in this section.

Sabadilla The standard symptoms of allergic rhinitis and hay fever, including runny nose, sneezing, and red, itchy eyes, are treated by the homeopathic medicine sabadilla, which is derived from the cevadilla seed. While taking it, also spend some time in the fresh air.

Wyethia Wyethia may benefit you if your allergy symptoms include an intense itching sensation on the soft palate of your mouth or itching behind your nose. Your symptoms may also include a dry feeling in your throat and nasal passages, even though your nose is running.

Arsenicum Album Arsenicum album, which is derived from arsenic trioxide, may be a useful medicine if your symptoms also include wheezing. Arsenicum is generally used as a cold medication. Symptoms that indicate a need for arsenicum include violent sneezing, a strong burning sensation in the nasal passages, headache, coughing, and constricted air passages with some wheezing. Other indications of the need for arsenicum include experiencing some relief from coughing after drinking warm liquid, and a burning sensation in the chest.

Euphrasia Euphrasia is derived from the herb commonly called eyebright, and it is useful in treating allergic rhinitis that is accompanied by an excessively runny nose and a loose cough, as well as burning tears. Generally, the runny nose is worse in the morning and when lying down, and the cough is also worse in the daytime.

When using any of these medicines, first try one dose and wait for a reaction. Generally, you will be provided with dosage information by your homeopathic medicine supplier, or the standard dose will be indicated on the container. If taking a dose of the medicine causes your symptoms to improve, wait until the symptoms return before you take any more. If your symptoms do not improve after four hours, take another dose and wait an additional four hours.

Use a homeopathic medicine no more than three times per day, and for no more than a week. If you do not experience an improvement in your symptoms by this time, you have most likely chosen the wrong medicine. Talk with your supplier about the symptoms the medicine is supposed to treat, and consider trying another one. It is also advisable to consult with a homeopathic physician.

If your symptoms become more severe and especially if your breathing becomes labored, consult a physician immediately. And if additional symptoms appear, and they are uncomfortable, it is best to discontinue using the medicine.

Keep in mind that homeopathic medicine is actually treating your illness with a remedy that causes similar symptoms to those you are experiencing. Again, this is based on the philosophy of treating like with like, to restore balance to the system. If you experience a new set of symptoms, you have probably not chosen the correct remedy since, under normal circumstances, homeopathic remedies work quickly. Keep your practitioner apprised of these changes.

While you know your own symptoms much better than anyone else, and can experiment with homeopathic medicines as you desire, a practitioner can make all the difference in getting your treatment on track.

Macrobiotics

The macrobiotic approach to healing is primarily dietary; however, this diet is based on a philosophy emphasizing the relationship of humankind with nature and the universe. When we are living in harmony with nature, the result is health and happiness. When we're out of harmony, through our diet, lifestyle, and thoughts, the result is sickness. Thus, healing is a matter of getting back in touch with nature and restoring our relationship. Macrobiotic practitioners not only prescribe diet and lifestyle changes, but also employ a range of natural treatments, many of which are based on plants and herbs, such as ginger.

According to macrobiotic theory, we can achieve harmony with nature through diet and thought. From this belief comes the macrobiotic diet. The right food helps to bring our cells, blood, thoughts, and emotions into balance. And through the thought process, we learn what actions need to be taken to maintain this harmony, as well as develop a positive attitude toward nature.

The macrobiotic diet is based on the Chinese medicine concepts of yin and yang, which were described in Chapter 2. Good health is based on a balance of yin and yang elements, with some foods having yin qualities and others having yang qualities. Illness, including allergic rhinitis and hay fever, results from having an imbalance that results from too much of one or the other. Much of this imbalance is due to poor diet.

According to macrobiotics, yang foods include eggs and meat, as well as salt. Yin foods include sugar, certain fruits, and vegetables. An excess of any of these can lead to an imbalance of yin and yang. Allergic rhinitis may be one consequence.

The Macrobiotic Diet A common misconception of the macrobiotic diet is that it is complicated; however it is really relatively simple. It includes basic elements that must be present in every meal, with options in terms of what specific foods can be eaten, as well as additional foods that can be eaten on a less regular basis. In a macrobiotic diet, at least half of each meal must consist of whole grains, including whole wheat, brown rice, barley, corn, and others. Vegetables should be approximately one third of every meal, with some of them cooked and some eaten raw. Daily intake should also include cooked beans, such as chickpeas and lentils, as well as seaweed. A small amount of soup, seasoned with natural flavorings like tamari, a kind of soy sauce, should also be consumed daily. Natural teas and some coffee are allowed as beverages.

While this is the basic regimen, the macrobiotic diet also includes guidelines for cooking food, condiments that can be used, and even how the food should be chewed to enhance digestion. Other lifestyle guidelines are also followed by macrobiotics followers. An attitude of gratefulness and friendliness is recommended, for example, as are daily walks to enjoy nature.

The basic macrobiotic diet varies little, regardless of the illness for which healing is desired. The reason is that macrobiotics is meant to be a lifestyle, with diet being an important component, rather than a fad adopted for a few days as a means of making symptoms disappear. Followers of macrobiotics believe that not only will this diet rid the system of toxins that are causing symptoms like mucus buildup and sneezing, but the diet will also keep illness at bay and restore peace of mind and a sense of calm.

Treating Allergic Rhinitis and Hay Fever with Macrobiotics   Allergic rhinitis and hay fever are viewed as the result of excessive eating, particularly of rich foods, as well as chemical additives. The foods that are viewed as the most likely culprits in causing this condition are yin foods such as dairy products, especially cold milk. Fruit and sugar can also contribute to the problem.

When food builds up in the system the body becomes so overburdened that it begins to store the excess, rather than eliminating it. This excess can come in various forms including mucus, which accumulates in the sinuses. Allergens like pollen are also yin. Because the body already has an overabundance of yin, when it comes into contact with pollen the mucous membranes react by trying to discharge it. The result is sneezing, runny nose, and other allergic rhinitis symptoms.

While a strict macrobiotic diet would be a practitioner's first recommendation, to allow the system to detoxify itself and regain balance without being bombarded by more excessive eating, a range of other remedies would also be used. These would include a compress of lotus root and ginger, made and applied in a manner similar to the compresses described in the homeopathy section in this chapter.

Working with Macrobiotics   Learn as much as possible about macrobiotics as you evaluate how it might be helpful for you. Macrobiotic practitioners are available in many communities, as are classes through organizations and adult education programs. You may even be able to find a local group of individuals who have chosen a macrobiotic way of life. A wide range of books on macrobiotics is also available. Macrobiotics is a complement to Oriental medicine, including acupuncture and acupressure, as well as relaxation techniques such as meditation.

If you decide to get serious about a macrobiotic diet, talk with your medical doctor. If you have a condition like diabetes, you'll need to make sure the dietary restrictions will not interfere with your condition.

Meditation

Meditation is widely recognized as an excellent way to relieve stress by creating a sense of inner peace. And when you feel an allergic reaction coming on, or are in the midst of one, creating a sense of peace and relaxation will also calm the immune system. Scientific evidence supports this theory, as research has shown that meditation can lower blood pressure as well as heart and respiratory rates. A wide range of meditation techniques are being taught, most of which are based on Eastern religions where meditation is used in creating peace of mind. Regardless of which technique you choose to learn, it's the result—the ability to create your own state of calmness—that counts.

The best approach to meditation is to learn a technique and then practice it on a daily basis, even if it is for only a few minutes every day, generally in the morning. The result of this practice is a sense of calm that will stay with you during the remainder of the day. Additionally, with practice you will be able to use your meditation technique to help achieve calm when you suddenly find yourself in a stressful situation, especially one in which you might be more susceptible to allergens.

Here is an example of a meditation technique to use on a daily basis and when you are threatened by an allergic reaction:

1. Go into a quiet room. Sit in an upright position in a straight-back chair, or lie flat on your back on the floor.

2. Close your eyes and consciously relax your body from the top of your head to the bottom of your feet.

3. Inhale through your nose, listening to your breath as it enters your body. Exhale through your mouth, mentally observing the breath as it leaves. Continue this observation of your breathing. It

may help to say a word or phrase such as "I am calm" each time you exhale.

4. As you go through this process, thoughts will flow in and out of your mind. Acknowledge them, but don't get too caught up in them. Let them pass out of your mind as you exhale. Focus on your breath.

5. After around fifteen minutes, open your eyes and sit quietly. Think about how calm and powerful you feel. You have achieved this calmness on your own, without waiting for it to be given to you, and you can achieve it anytime you want by using the same technique.

6. As you continue to practice, you will become more adept at relaxing yourself, and you will relax at a deeper level.

A wide range of books are available that teach meditation techniques. Classes are also available through community education programs, holistic education centers, yoga or zen centers, the YMCA or YWCA, or any number of similar resources. Generally, the cost is minimal. A class can be particularly helpful if you haven't tried meditation before, because a supportive leader is available to provide guidance and answer any questions.

You may see the results of meditation soon, if not immediately, after your first practice session. But sometimes obtaining results takes a longer time. Meditation is a great practice to get into because it provides you with an ability to become more calm and centered in all areas of your life. And it's also helpful when used in conjunction with other practices such as yoga.

Naturopathy

Naturopathic practitioners view allergic rhinitis and hay fever and asthma as being similar both in terms of the factors that cause them and the recommended treatments, and in many instances, allergy is a trigger for asthma. The naturopathic approach to allergic rhinitis and hay fever will be discussed here, and asthma will be discussed in more depth in Chapter 6.

Naturopaths look to two major causes in determining the factors that lead to the symptoms of allergic rhinitis and hay fever. The first of these causes is food allergies that result in symptoms such as sneezing and congestion. These symptoms can be immediate, and possibly related to sensitivities to foods such as fish, eggs, nuts, and shellfish; or the symptoms can be delayed and more likely the result of allergies to foods like wheat, chocolate, milk products, and food coloring. A low degree of stomach acidity is another factor recognized by naturopaths in the development of allergic rhinitis and hay fever, with food staying in the stomach longer and creating imbalances that lead to allergy.

Food allergy and a low degree of stomach acidity are also associated with asthma, as is exposure to food additives, like artificial dyes and preservatives. This is discussed in Chapter 6.

Treating Allergic Rhinitis and Hay Fever with Naturopathy The primary approach to treating allergic rhinitis and hay fever is dietary. Naturopaths will often recommend a vegetarian diet, avoiding all meat, fish, dairy products, and eggs. Drinking water is limited to spring water, with avoidance of coffee, soda, and other stimulants, as well as sugar and salt. The naturopath's allergy diet includes unlimited amounts of vegetables, including lettuce, broccoli, celery, beets, cucumber, and most beans except soy and green beans. Restricted amounts of potatoes are allowed, with most fruits except apples and citrus, and very restricted amounts of grains.

The benefit of this diet is that it eliminates the allergens that are being consumed through the food, resulting in a gradual detoxification.

Naturopaths will also recommend the use of botanical medicines in treating allergic rhinitis and hay fever. These medicines include Ephedra, a natural remedy used for thousands of years in treating allergy symptoms. The Ephedra plant contains components that act as antiinflammatory and antiallergy agents; a synthetic compound made from Ephedra, called ephedrine, is used in many prescription medications for asthma and hay fever. The usefulness of Ephedra diminishes if it is used repeatedly over time, and it is often supplemented by other herbs like licorice, as well as vitamin C, vitamin B_6, and other nutritional supplements.

Skullcap is another botanical medicine often used by naturopaths in treating allergic rhinitis and hay fever. It has an antiinflammatory action, and inhibits allergy symptoms by combatting the effects of the histamines. Angelica, onions, and garlic are also among the herbal medicines that a naturopath will draw upon in treating allergy.

As noted in Chapter 3, naturopaths take a holistic approach to treating allergy. Diet modification, exercise, and preventive measures like avoidance of what you know to be allergens will be important aspects of your treatment. Detoxification, to rid your system of the allergy-causing toxins, will also be important. Herbal remedies may, or may not, be part of your treatment.

Talk with your medical doctor about your naturopath's plan for treating your allergic rhinitis and hay fever. If you are currently receiving desensitization injections or taking antihistamines, these treatments may not be compatible with some of the herbal remedies that may be recommended by your naturopath. Discuss the implications with both individuals, particularly potential emergency situations that can result from allergy symptoms. You may be able to use both approaches in tandem, or you may have to make a choice. In any case, don't place your health and well-being in jeopardy.

Nutrition

Allergic rhinitis and hay fever are generally believed to be caused by food allergies, and a diet heavy in preservatives and other additives, and animal fat. Working with a nutritionist to develop a balanced diet may help to lower the oversensitivity that contributes to allergic reaction.

Many nutritionists think that specific foods can contribute to allergic rhinitis and hay fever. For example, if you have an allergy to birch pollen, you may react to foods like hazelnuts, since birch and hazel belong to the same family. Consuming yeast, which is found in alcoholic and brewed beverages, and bread, can contribute to allergic rhinitis if yeast is an allergen for you. Generally, allergic rhinitis symptoms will not appear immediately; instead they may begin many hours after the food is consumed and digested. Thus, it is often difficult to see the association between what you have eaten and the appearance of symptoms.

Your nutritionist is not going to create a miracle diet to rid you of all allergic rhinitis and hay fever symptoms. However, as an allergic person, your body is overreacting to substances in the environment, like pollen and mold. If you are not eating a balanced diet, and are consuming prepared foods that are high in preservatives, you are placing yourself at a further disadvantage by loading your system with toxins. A balanced diet gives you an advantage in standing up to the allergens that you breathe.

A nutritionist will most likely provide you with guidelines for a balanced diet that suits your lifestyle while also helping you to avoid allergic rhinitis and hay fever symptoms. You may want to consider trying the elimination diet, described in Chapter 3, to discover if the use of stimulants or certain foods is also contributing to your symptoms. Most likely, you won't know until you go through this process and test out the foods you are accustomed to eating.

Physicians are increasingly aware of the importance of a good diet and often refer their patients to nutritionists. In any case, make sure your physician is aware that you are working with a nutritionist. Provide your nutritionist with a list of the substances you know you are allergic to so that, if necessary, related foods are placed on your forbidden-food list.

Psychotherapy

The connection between your emotions and allergy can be complicated. For example, while you may not be aware of it, your sniffling and sneezing can prevent you from being able to take an active role in life, or protect you from having to take risks. Your hay fever attacks can also prevent others from doing things they may want to do, like taking a camping trip, thereby giving you an added measure of control. And a few days of congestion can gain you a lot of sympathy. In other words, having allergy symptoms can be a negative means of getting what you want.

But aren't there healthier ways of getting our needs met? Yes, but the only way to find out where allergy fits in with our psychological makeup is by working with a therapist to find out where this connection started, and how to replace it with more positive behaviors. This may mean going back into your early childhood and delving into where your conflicts, and resulting behaviors, developed. Somewhere during the process of growing up, you may have discovered that getting sick got you what you wanted. Or you may have learned to associate certain people, or situations, with sneezing and congestion. Have you ever been in an argument with someone and suddenly found yourself debilitated by nasal congestion and violent sneezing?

Psychotherapy not only helps you sort out your past and see how it is still affecting you in the present, it is also a way of discovering new, and healthier, behaviors. New ways of coping with stress. Techniques for keeping yourself relaxed, and less edgy, during hay fever season. Strategies for saying what you mean, and getting what you want, without having to get sick first.

Psychotherapy can take some time. Make sure you work with a therapist with whom you are comfortable, and who has experience in working with clients who experience physical complaints. You might also consider a group therapy situation, perhaps with others like yourself who have allergic rhinitis or hay fever. In a group, you'll learn from others who have had similar experiences with allergy and emotions, and gain support as you deal with your own condition.

You may find that your hay fever is just hay fever. However, psychotherapy can still help you to adjust to your condition and effectively deal with your feelings before you set yourself up for symptoms that might otherwise be avoidable.

Reflexology

In addition to promoting relaxation and stress reduction, reflexology can also be helpful in treating allergic rhinitis by strengthening areas of the body that are most susceptible to this condition. One of these areas is the sinuses. Pollens that cause hay fever can irritate the membranes of the sinuses and cause them to swell, which results in discomfort. Air pollution and colds can also irritate the sinuses.

Reflexology treats the sinuses in two ways. First, it helps to keep the membranes in this region healthy and free of debris. Reflexology can also be used to relieve allergy symptoms in this area by relieving congestion and unclogging the air passages.

The reflex points for the sinuses are on both the hands and feet. On the hands, the points are located at the top joints and knuckles of both the thumbs and fingers. On the feet, the nasal passages and sinus points are on the top joints and knuckles of the toes. These areas, on both the hands and feet, include the tips, pads, and nails. The points on the left side correspond with the left side of the sinuses, and vice versa.

When working the sinus reflex points on the hand, start with the top joint on the thumb. Grasp it between your other thumb, index finger, and middle finger, and press firmly, using a gentle rolling motion. Move from the thumb to each finger of the hand. When you have worked each digit, go through the hand again, this time pressing each one slightly harder. Go through this sequence seven times, then give the thumb and each finger a gentle twist. Repeat this whole sequence on the other hand.

When working the reflex points of the feet, place the index and middle finger of one hand on the toe that you are going to work. Place the thumb of the other hand on the bottom of the toe, so that you are holding the foot with both hands. Press firmly, with a rolling motion. The sequence should begin with the big toe, then moving on the other toes, one at a time. Repeat this action seven times, slightly increasing the pressure during each round. After the seventh round, give each toe a slight twist.

While a reflexology practitioner is best qualified to treat your allergy symptoms, you can learn to use reflexology techniques on your own, or with a partner. When applying reflexology, you can work the general areas where the reflex points are located, rather than trying to locate the specific point. Massage these areas gently but firmly, working an area on one hand or foot, then moving to the same area on the other hand or foot. As you press into an area, inhale slowly and deeply. Then exhale as you release the pressure.

Shiatsu

Shiatsu, discussed briefly in Chapter 2, is a form of therapeutic massage that originated in Japan. It differs from holistic massage in that, while it does promote relaxation, it is based on techniques that are aimed at providing relief for specific symptoms, including various forms of chronic pain and temporary illness. Shiatsu is also useful in treating the symptoms of allergic rhinitis and hay fever.

Shiatsu combines diagnosis and therapy in that a trained practitioner is able to use his or her hands both in detecting abnormalities in the skin or muscles and make decisions as to what form of treatment to apply. While treatments are applied accordingly, shiatsu is also holistic in that it promotes the health of the entire body.

Shiatsu is based on a belief in *chi*, which is a vital force that flows through all the connected channels, or meridians, throughout the body. Each of these meridians is connected to an organ or to an aspect of the personality. The *chi* associated with a meridian can be contacted along specific points—the same points that are used in acupressure and acupuncture. When your health is at its best, the energy flowing along the paths between the meridians of your body is balanced. But when you are not feeling well, due to stress, illness, an accumulation of toxins, or some other condition, the flow becomes imbalanced. There is too much *chi* in some areas, and not enough in others. An overabundance of *chi* is referred to as *jitsu*, and a deficiency is called *kyo*.

With the stresses of modern life, the pollution in our environment, as well as the additives in our food, most of us are walking around with systems that are at least somewhat out of balance, regardless of how well we feel. As these imbalances continue untreated, however, the result may be ailments like allergy.

Treating Your Allergic Rhinitis and Hay Fever with Shiatsu The instruments of the shiatsu practitioner are the hands, and he or she is trained to use every part of the hand in applying different types of pressure. The thumb is particularly important in applying pressure to specific points of the body. How pressure is applied, and with which part of the hand, is a decision the practitioner makes based on the diagnosis of your condition, the meridian to which the pressure is being applied, and the desired effect. Unlike holistic massage, no oils are used in shiatsu, and the person receiving shiatsu is not nude but instead wears comfortable, loose clothing.

Shiatsu is useful in treating the symptoms of allergy and other illnesses. However, because it also corrects imbalances in the system, qualified practitioners may cure your condition. The key word here is "qualified." Being able to identify the various meridians of the body, make a diagnosis, and perform the needed corrective action is the result of years of training, both in Oriental medicine as well as specific shiatsu techniques.

Although shiatsu is an art, you can learn a few basic techniques that you can use with a partner in getting relief for some of your own symptoms, and even practice on yourself. The following is a technique you can use on someone else, or teach someone to use on you.

The recipient should lie on his or her left side, with the right leg crossed over the left one. The head should be slightly elevated. The giver then massages the medulla oblongata area, on the lower part of the back of the head, as well as on the back of the neck. This action causes the blood vessels in the nasal membrane to contract, thus relieving congestion to allow breathing through the nose.

Another technique for treating head congestion begins with the receiver lying on his or her back. The giver then gently uses the thumbs to massage the frontal meridian, which is located in the center of the face, just above the nose. Following this action, pressure with index and middle fingers of both hands is gently applied at both sides of the nose.

Chest congestion and cough can be relieved by shiatsu techniques applied to the back of the shoulders. The receiver lies on his or her stomach. The giver presses with one hand on the right shoulder blade, while laying the length of the thumb of the other hand along the top of the right shoulder. The giver then presses gently outward, from the neck to the notch in the shoulder joint. This is then repeated on the other shoulder.

Another technique for relieving chest congestion requires the giver to sit back and place his or her feet on the top of the receiver's shoulders. The giver then presses gently in a treading motion.

Working with a Shiatsu Practitioner   As discussed earlier, to gain the full benefit from shiatsu, work with a qualified shiatsu practitioner. You can most likely find individuals who practice this specialty by looking at a listing of massage therapists in your area, or by checking at a local health food store or holistic health center. And as you contact practitioners, ask about their training and certification.

Your practitioner will learn more about your condition by giving you a complete shiatsu treatment, beginning with your back, then moving on to the hips, the back of the legs, the back of the shoulders, front of the shoulders, head and face, arms and hands, front of the legs, and then chest and abdomen. During this process, he or she will locate various meridians and make diagnoses concerning where the *chi* is in overabundance or deficiency. Treatments will begin from here, and each will last between thirty minutes and one hour.

While shiatsu is relatively risk free, there are still a few cautions. You should not receive it if you are suffering from a sprain, or a whiplash, or have a herniated disk. It should also be avoided if you are pregnant, have a contagious disease, or internal conditions like appendicitis, ulcers, intestinal obstructions, cancer, or leukemia. View shiatsu as primarily a means of relieving your allergic rhinitis and hay fever symptoms and continue with the medications you may be receiving from your physician. You may also want to have your physician check your general physical condition and warn you of any risk factors before you undertake shiatsu.

Your shiatsu practitioner will most likely do more than provide you with shiatsu treatments. He or she may recommend breathing exercises as well as a balanced diet. Physical exercise, using complementary approaches such as yoga, is often recommended, as is meditation.

Visualization

When you visualize, you use the power of your imagination to achieve the outcome you are seeking—in this case, increased relaxation, and less sensitivity to pollen and other allergens that set off your allergy symptoms.

Visualization begins with relaxation, because you can't focus your mind until you have cleared the chaos out of the way. Meditation techniques can help with this. Once your mind is relaxed, you start introducing desired outcomes gradually, through pictures. A strong immune system might look like a rose that starts as a tiny bud that gets larger and stronger until it blossoms. Or you might visualize yourself sitting on a beach, smelling the sea breeze, listening to the waves, and breathing in clean, allergen-free air. Visualize yourself as a person who is in charge of his or her reactions to the environment, and not a victim.

Here is a visualization you can practice on your own:

1. Find a quiet place with no distractions. Sit upright in a straight-back chair. Place both feet on the floor and relax your hands at your side.

2. Inhale deeply, and feel yourself blow out all of your stressful thoughts and feelings as you exhale.

3. While you concentrate on your breathing, consciously relax every muscle in your body, beginning with your facial muscles, moving down to the chest, the arms and hands, the upper legs, lower legs, and feet.

4. Choose a visualization like one of those described above, with your immune system as a rose, for example. Or visualize yourself in a potentially threatening situation, but symptom free. Or just

visualize yourself in a comfortable, happy place, feeling calm and comfortable and loved.

Visualization helps you in many ways. First of all, it is a way of training yourself to experience positive, empowered reactions to situations that normally cause you to have allergic symptoms. Visualization also helps you to relax, and relaxation is one of your best defenses when faced with allergens. Use visualization to harness your own natural healing powers.

There are a great many books available that teach visualization techniques. Churches with a metaphysical orientation may offer visualization workshops, as do holistic education and training centers. In a workshop, you will learn techniques for relaxing, which is the key to effective visualization, as well as how to create and focus on images of health and enlightenment. Also, in a workshop you are surrounded by the positive energy of the people around you, and this energy will boost your efforts as you practice using visualization techniques.

It takes years of practice to create the negative images we all carry around, and counteracting them with positive images will also take time and practice. Don't be surprised if you are uncomfortable with the process at first, and even unable to create a visualization at first. Focus on learning to relax, then begin imagining situations from your past in which you felt secure and happy. Once you teach yourself to relax and create positive visualizations, you can begin targeting your visualizations toward new situations you want to create in your life.

CHAPTER FIVE

Juvenile Allergies

It has been estimated that one of every five children who visits a pediatrician is there because of some type of allergy. Children suffer from many of the same allergies as adults, with many of the same symptoms. Juvenile allergies often begin with reactions to certain foods, especially milk, and it is not uncommon for a child to suffer from a range of allergies, from hay fever to eczema. Yet, allergic children often differ in the way they respond to an allergen—two children can be exposed to pollen and one will sneeze while the other one wheezes.

The treatment options for juvenile allergies are in many instances the same as those for adults, though with some modifications. In this chapter, natural treatments are discussed in terms of conditions that include allergic rhinitis and hay fever, skin allergy, and food allergy.

THE ROOTS OF JUVENILE ALLERGIES

Children may develop allergies for a variety of reasons. Heredity is a factor—if someone is allergic, there is a good chance that at least one of their children will also be allergic. Exposure to chemicals and environmental pollutants that the mother has touched, eaten, or inhaled may also increase a child's potential to become allergic. Breast-feeding may be a factor, with the mother passing on antigens during the infant's first few months out of the womb. Childhood illness can make the immune system vulnerable. Medications like hydrocortisone can also cause an allergic reaction, which is a good reason to explore natural medicine for treating your child's allergies.

A child's immune system is much more sensitive than that of an adult. Because of this sensitivity, children are much more likely to acquire various allergies; even infants come down with diaper rashes, sniffles, coughs, and irritability, all of which can be caused by allergies.

What is important is that the allergies be recognized at an early stage, and treated. While the experts disagree as to whether or not allergies are "curable," early intervention can certainly make your child's life, and your life, much easier, and minimize any further damage that might occur.

How Do I Know if It's Allergy?

The immune systems of children are in the development stages, and they are not always effective in fighting off illness. Consequently, children are often sick. And when they are around each other, they often take turns passing various colds and viruses to each other and, at times, to their parents. So how do you know when these symptoms are caused by an allergy?

Allergy symptoms are chronic, meaning they occur often and stick around for a while. They're not like colds or viruses that run their course and then disappear. Additionally, the symptoms are, as a group, fairly predictable. The areas affected by juvenile allergies, along with symptoms, are listed below:

Skin—An itchy rash that may look like hives; raised and red weals; or a patchy or raw and oozing red, scaly rash like eczema.

Nose—A runny nose with a clear, watery discharge (rather than the heavier discharge that results from a cold), usually accompanied by sneezing. An allergic runny nose can go on for weeks, and usually becomes red and itchy.

Eyes—Red, itchy, and runny eyes, with swollen lids.

Ears—Itchy, and possibly dripping, ears. The ears often become plugged and the child may complain of difficulty in hearing.

Mouth—Itching, sometimes extreme, on the soft palate.

Chest—A continuous cough, often accompanied by shortness of breath and wheezing. This chest congestion can also result in pain in the ribs and chest muscles.

Gastrointestinal tract—Nausea, gas, bloating, diarrhea, and vomiting.

Juvenile allergies are in many cases not as easy to categorize as are adult allergies. For example, when coming into contact with an allergen, an adult with allergic rhinitis usually experiences a specific set of symptoms, while an adult with food allergies has another set. Children with allergies may respond to an allergen with a much wider range of symptoms, from sneezing to nausea to eczema. The reason for this range of symptoms is that a child's immune system is still developing, and is thus much more susceptible to the effects of allergens. Also, juvenile allergies often progress from food allergies to eczema to allergic rhinitis and then asthma; depending on how allergies are progressing, a child might exhibit any number of symptoms.

Food Allergies

One of a parent's greatest fears is milk allergy in an infant, which can lead to symptoms like diarrhea and vomiting, rashes, asthma, and a vulnerability to numerous infections. As with other allergies, it is difficult to predict where a child's milk allergy begins. However, factors include having a milk-allergic parent, being introduced to solid foods too early in life, and being bottle fed with cow's milk.

Many mothers with milk-allergic children had the same problem as children. This may be the result of a missing enzyme, namely lactase, the one that assists with milk digestion. Being fed cow's milk, rather than breast milk, may also be a factor. The mother passes on her own antibodies to the child, including an antibody that protects against foreign proteins. While cow's milk also contains antibodies, it is not as rich in the kinds of antibodies that humans need. Cow's milk also contains proteins that are difficult for the infant's stomach to break down effectively.

The link between food allergy and other allergies, in children, is both complex and, at this point, mysterious. Children are more susceptible to the food they eat. This can result in a range of symptoms that may include those normally associated with other types of allergy. Wheat and corn allergy, for example, can cause not only the more typical food allergy symptoms, such as nausea and diarrhea, but also skin irritations and nasal congestion. While a range of foods can cause allergic reactions in children, food additives are high on the list, including food dye, monosodium glutamate, and sulfites.

The best way to treat food allergies in children is through both avoidance of allergy-causing foods and adoption of a balanced diet using a minimal amount of food additives. This treatment begins with the elimination diet, described in Chapters 3 and 10. Symptoms of food allergy can also be treated with herbal remedies and relaxation techniques.

Skin Irritations

Why children develop skin irritations like hives and eczema is as much a mystery as why they develop any number of allergies. There are literally hundreds of potential substances, both natural and chemical, that can upset a child's immune system. Additionally, the actual appearance, location, and duration of skin irritations, particularly hives, are not at all predictable.

Ironically—and another point in favor of natural medicine—hives are often caused by medications that are supposed to provide a cure. Drugs like penicillin and other antibiotics, insulin, and sulfa can cause hives. Food additives and dyes are another cause, as are some foods like tomatoes, nuts, and shellfish. Hives can also be caused by infections, direct contact with chemical agents, and sudden changes in temperature.

The elimination diet, described in the Naturopathy section in Chapter 10, can be helpful in treating food-related allergies. Other natural treatments include lotions and creams that soothe itching and irritated skin without adding more chemicals to the system, as well as relaxation methods to lower the stress that can lead to skin irritation.

Allergic Rhinitis and Hay Fever

Allergic rhinitis and hay fever in children looks and acts very much like hay fever in adults. Symptoms appear during the peak pollen and mold seasons. In children, hay fever may look like a cold, with symptoms that never disappear. Hay fever is relatively easy to detect, with symptoms that include:

- Watery, clear nasal discharge
- Teary, itchy eyes
- Bouts of sneezing
- Breathing through the mouth
- Itchy ears and mouth
- Dark circles around the eyes during the peak seasons

To complicate matters, children are often unable to articulate how they are feeling, so they suffer without asking for help, and appear irritable, listless, and moody.

The medical establishment treats allergic rhinitis and hay fever through a wide range of options, including immunization, or allergy shots, and various medications such as antihistamines and decongestants. Immunization treats the cause of allergy through injecting the child with small amounts of allergens, with the goal of "wearing out" the allergy over time. Antihistamines and decongestants treat the symptoms of allergy, like sneezing and runny nose. These medications can have side effects, like dizziness and nervousness, though they are effective in providing instant relief.

Practitioners of natural medicine, however, view these approaches as contributing to the problem. Medications add more chemicals to the system, and these chemicals can be toxic, leading to other illnesses and allergies. Medications also interfere with the development of the body's natural defenses.

Treating only the physical symptoms of allergy is also neglecting the whole picture. Personality and emotions also play a role.

Juvenile Allergies and Emotions

Being allergic can present children with a whole range of pressures. They may feel different from other children at school, especially if allergies restrict them from being able to participate fully in school activities, or if they experience symptoms that make them look or feel different. Eczema, or red eyes and a runny nose, can set allergic children apart from peers, and draw stares and cruel comments. Similar problems can also arise at home. Medical expenditures and special equipment such as humidifiers may place a strain on the family budget. Parents and siblings may have to work extra hard to keep the house dust free. Vacations to places like a dude ranch may have to be avoided because of the one family member's allergies. The family pet may have to go. Even if reassured otherwise, allergic children often feel like outsiders in their own homes.

These situations can result in feelings of stress for allergic children, depending on how much emotional support they are receiving from the adults in their life. Being on guard against criticism, and being overly self-conscious, results in feelings of stress. When children experience stress, their immune system is also placed on alert, and the result is a greater tendency toward allergic reaction.

Conventional Medicine or Natural Medicine?

Children cannot make their own health decisions and are thus at the mercy of both their parents and the medical establishment. If you are the parent of an allergic child, this places you in the position of making decisions that may be, in every sense of the word, life or death. Many practitioners will tell you that medical doctors will prescribe medications such as cortisone, antihistamines, and decongestants that are much too strong for a child's system. On the other hand, medical doctors may tell you that your child's condition will not improve, and it may in fact become worse, without medications. Who do you trust?

Because of the possibility of anaphylactic shock, described in Chapter 3, it is recommended that you always have access to a medical doctor for your child's condition. This is especially true if your child's allergies are severe enough that anaphylactic shock is a possibility.

Don't experiment with treatments. Talk to your physician about the possibility of using natural treatment methods. Choose those that your child may benefit from but that will not interfere with his or her primary treatment. You can take advantage of the benefits of some natural remedies yet still avail your child of the wonders of modern medicine.

NATURAL TREATMENTS FOR CHILDHOOD ALLERGIES

Acupressure

Acupressure treatment can be highly beneficial for childhood allergies. With parental supervision, children can be taught to locate and use acupressure points that can give them relief of their allergy symptoms. While some of the exercises may be too complicated for children to undertake on their own, others are so simple that children can begin to relieve their own symptoms when their parents aren't around.

To investigate acupressure treatment for children, start with a practitioner who has experience in treating allergic children. You'll need to be involved at every step, observing and even assisting with each session so that you and your child work as a team in learning each exercise. Make sure your child understands the purpose of acupressure exercises and talks about how he or she feels during the exercises as well as afterward. If pain or any other negative effects are reported, the practitioner will need to make adjustments.

The cost of an acupressure session for a child is much the same as that for an adult. Most practitioners will schedule regular sessions at first, to monitor progress, with sporadic sessions thereafter.

Some of the acupressure exercises useful for adult allergies may not be as comfortable for young children because they are more sensitive to the firm pressure often required for maximum results. Make sure you discuss your concerns with your practitioner, and also report any discomfort that your child exhibits.

Affirmations

Children quickly learn, through experience, that when they come into contact with certain allergens, allergy symptoms will follow. Their bodies get ready for the attack. Experience is also compounded by what they hear from their parents and other adults. If you had allergies as a child, you may remember your mother saying things like "Stay away from cats. You'll start sneezing and wheezing" or "Don't drink any milk. You'll get sick." While these warnings helped to keep you from becoming symptomatic, they also turned into messages that you internalized, and began playing for yourself.

Children should not be encouraged to expose themselves to allergens. However, they can be encouraged not to think of themselves as victims—as sick people—and instead to focus on getting better. Affirmations can also help when children are in the midst of an allergic reaction, producing a calming effect that in turn calms the immune system. Adults can help with this process by creating simple affirmations that focus on the positive, and practicing them with their children.

Here are a few affirmations to use with allergic children.

- I don't have to be afraid.
- I am strong and healthy.
- I am getting better every day.
- I can take care of my allergies and still have fun.

Using affirmations can become a game, with parents and children working together to create them. Writing them down on sheets of paper that can be hung on the bedroom wall, and even drawing pictures to illustrate them, can help. Try practicing affirmations before school, maybe during breakfast, and again before bedtime.

Aromatherapy

Aromatherapy, described in depth in Chapter 4, is an excellent natural treatment for children with allergies. An aroma lamp, for example, can be placed in a child's room, permeating the room with aromas that promote health and help to quell the symptoms of allergy. While you should avoid placing an open flame in a child's room, lamps that use light bulbs can both be fun and serve as a night light. Children love smelling the fresh fragrances. Lotions and salves based on essential oils can help to heal the effects of eczema.

Children have a very sensitive sense of smell. In fact, within a few weeks after birth, a baby can recognize and respond to the odor of its mother. Scents bond a mother and child, and mothers are often able to detect when a child is ill from a change in his or her scent. Fragrances can help in developing creativity, enhancing intelligence, and encouraging a positive attitude. Fragrances can also be used in healing childhood illnesses.

Aromatherapy helps to reduce the effects of allergies caused by inhalants in much the same way as with adults. The aromas from the essential oils counteract the effects of inhalants by stimulating the relief-giving and health-enhancing neurotransmitters of the central nervous system. Salves also may relieve eczema.

You can visit an aromatherapist to discuss your child's specific allergies, and get help in deciding which essential oils might be most helpful in relieving allergy symptoms. As a rule of thumb, children's systems are more sensitive than adults, and they will not require as many drops of whatever oil you are using. Also, some oils may be too strong for children and an aromatherapist can tell you which ones to avoid. You may find some of this same information in a comprehensive book on aromatherapy.

The essential oils that children seem to respond to best include tangerine, orange, cinnamon, honey oil, and vanilla. Placing one of these scents in a child's room will promote calm, a sense of well-being, and general good health. You may want to read your child a special story as these scents permeate the room.

The following are suggested applications of aromatherapy for relieving childhood allergies:

Congestion   Essential oils used in an aroma lamp can relieve congestion by acting as an expectorant and decongestant. The essential oils to use include eucalyptus, mountain pine, myrtle, naiouli, and lemon. Just two drops of these oils, which is about half the adult dose, is enough.

Sensitive Skin Sensitive, easily irritated skin is more susceptible to allergic reactions. To keep your child's skin healthy and supple, add a few drops of essential oils to his or her bathwater. A good bath mix includes five drops of Roman chamomile and two drops of neroli, mixed with a few tablespoons of honey and bran.

Stomach Ailments The upset stomach and cramps that often result from allergy to milk and other foods can sometimes be relieved by using the essential oils of fennel or coriander. For children, use one or two drops, with honey if desired, diluted in water or warm tea.

Keep in mind that essential oils can have toxic side effects, and these effects can be much more pronounced in children. Always keep essential oils out of the reach of young children.

Botanical Medicine

The use of herbs in treating childhood allergies, as described in Chapter 4, can be very helpful. This is especially true when herbal preparations are used to relieve the congestion and mucus production that often accompanies an allergic reaction, the nausea and diarrhea that can follow a food allergy, and the hives and eczema that are produced by a skin allergy. The botanical medicine approach to childhood allergies is similar to that of adult allergies in that the starting place for treatment is through detoxification of the system to rid it of impurities, followed by the treatment of specific symptoms, and then strengthening the weakened areas.

Most of the common herbs are relatively mild, and are relatively safe when used externally or in mild teas. When using herbs internally, children require special precautions. Treating adult symptoms may require a large amount of an herb, but this is not true for children. In fact, children need much less of an herb to be affected by it. Some herbs, particularly those with a spicy or hot taste, can be distasteful and upsetting to children. Herbs may trigger new allergies. Furthermore, any potential toxic side effect of an herb may be greatly magnified when given to a child.

When working with children, use herbs carefully. Greatly dilute the standard adult dose. Don't use them internally without working with a practitioner who has experience in treating children. Also keep in mind that the use of herbs may affect the medical treatment your child may be receiving, especially since many medications are derived from herbs. Consult your pediatrician to make sure he or she is aware of this treatment and supports it.

In greatly diluted amounts, children can benefit from the use of herbs in treating their allergy symptoms. Herbs stimulate a child's own natural defenses and further strengthen the system without adding artificial chemicals, alcohol, sugar, food dye, and other additives to his or her system at the same time. An herbal preparation can be used as a mild antacid to soothe an upset stomach. Herbs with antibiotic properties may relieve an ear infection. Carminative herbs, such as might be obtained in a mild peppermint tea, can relieve intestinal pain. Emollient herbs may provide a gentle treatment for an outbreak of eczema. A poultice with mustard oil or eucalyptus might relieve the congestion and mucus production that result from, for example, exposure to the neighbor's cat.

Herbs may also have strengthening and restorative effects on children. They can be used to make the respiratory system healthier, helping your child to stand up to the effects of allergic reactions, as well as related conditions such as asthma. Herbs can also build up the digestive system to help in reducing the food allergy symptoms, or even prevent them. Herbs that purify the blood can lessen the effects of all allergic reactions, including skin conditions.

When treating your child with herbs, there are a few rules of thumb to keep in mind. First and foremost, as mentioned previously, work with a practitioner, with the approval of your pediatrician. Use greatly reduced amounts of each herb. If your practitioner has recommended using an herb internally, and your child complains about the taste of the herb, do not force it on him or her. Try chopping it up in a spoonful of honey or peanut butter. Watch closely for any reactions, as well as improvement. If your child's symptoms worsen, discontinue use immediately and seek medical attention if your child seems to be having a reaction of any severity. And if you don't see any improvement in your child's condition within a few days, check with your practitioner. Unless the herb was intended to strengthen and nurture your child's natural defenses gradually, it may not be working.

Botanical medicine should not be used with aromatherapy or with homeopathy because they all rely on herbs, and the approaches may interfere with each other.

Here are a few herbal treatments for juvenile allergy that you can try at home.

Congestion Congestion and mucus production can sometimes be relieved by a compress using ginger. Mix a few drops of a tincture of ginger, which you can purchase from a health food store, with four tablespoons of whole wheat flour and enough water to make a paste. Spread it on a piece of cotton cloth, and then lay it over your child's chest. Leave it on for at least an hour.

Skin Irritations Comfrey comes from the root and leaves of the comfrey plant, and is known to promote the growth of cells and soothe skin inflammations. It is especially good for treating your child's eczema. To make a salve of comfrey, follow these steps:

1. Rub about two ounces of comfrey herb between your hands and place it in a glass jar. Add two ounces of either olive or sesame oil and seal the jar.
2. Shake the jar every day for at least two weeks.
3. Strain the contents through cheesecloth to remove the herb fragments. The result is an herbal oil.
4. Place this strained oil in a pot and simmer it slowly for a few hours.
5. In a can placed in boiling water, melt about an ounce of beeswax and then pour it into the oil.
6. Simmer the mixture until it has the consistency of salve. To check the consistency, take out a teaspoonful of the hot salve and let it cool in the refrigerator for a moment. Test it with your finger to make sure it is spreadable.
7. Add a few drops of vitamin E oil.
8. Pour the thickened oil into a small jar.

Rub the salve directly on dermatitis, hives, or eczema, and use it as needed to reduce symptoms, including itchiness. The best time to apply the salve is before your child goes to bed.

Upset Stomach A ginger tea can be effective in treating the symptoms of food allergy, including indigestion and gas. To make a quart of ginger tea, follow these directions:

1. Grate two inches of fresh gingerroot.
2. Place it in a teapot.
3. Boil one quart of water, and then pour it over the ginger.
4. Cover the teapot and let it steep at least fifteen minutes.
5. Drink it warm or cool.

Serve the ginger tea to your child a few times per day, or until the symptoms disappear.

Homeopathy

Homeopathy, discussed in some depth in Chapters 2 and 4, can work well when applied to childhood allergies. Childhood allergies, as with adult allergies, are caused by an imbalanced immune system: the immune system is recognizing harmless substances as allergens.

Children are especially sensitive to medications. Excessive use of medications can worsen the situations and further interfere with the natural ability for self-healing. Not only do symptoms return but immune system development can be slowed down by the presence of drugs. Also, medications, including those used to treat allergies, as well as antibiotics, only cover symptoms and short-circuit the healing process. Medications also contain chemicals that can cause side effects that can in turn be a factor in causing symptoms.

If illness is allowed to take its course, the child's natural defenses are often capable of fighting it off while also becoming stronger in the process. Using homeopathic remedies for childhood allergies provides that extra stimulus the child's defenses need to complete the healing cycle, with natural-based medicines that work with, and enhance, immune system development.

Applying Homeopathy to Juvenile Allergies As with adults, homeopathic remedies for children are chosen to match as closely as possible the symptoms the child is exhibiting. Again, the treatment is based on choosing a single medicine that mimics the symptoms. As with other homeopathic treatments, children are given only one medicine at a time.

The following are major homeopathic remedies used for juvenile allergies, arranged by allergy group. Keep in mind that you can obtain and use these medicines on your own. However, children are more sensitive than adults and you will want to use some caution in applying them. These cautions are discussed later in this section. As with all therapies for children, always check first with your pediatrician before giving your child any remedy.

Respiratory Allergies As with other homeopathic remedies, those used in treating a child's respiratory system mimic the group of symptoms that the child is experiencing. These symptoms will include not only the standard allergy indicators but also symptoms like restlessness, irritability, and inability to sleep.

Sabadilla, from the cevadilla seed, is a common remedy for allergic rhinitis and hay fever when the symptoms include runny nose, sneezing, and red, itchy eyes. Wyethia may be needed when symptoms include an intense itching sensation in the soft palate of the mouth and behind the nose. Symptoms indicating a need for Wyethia also include a runny nose, but with a dry feeling in the throat and nasal passages.

Arsenicum album, from arsenic trioxide, may also be given for childhood allergies, especially when the symptoms include wheezing, violent sneezing, a burning sensation in the nasal passages, headache, coughing, and constricted air passages. Arsenicum is also indicated if your child's coughing is somewhat relieved after drinking a warm liquid or if he or she feels a burning sensation in the chest. Euphrasia, derived from the herb, eyebright, is used when the allergy symptoms also include an excessively runny nose and a loose cough, accompanied by burning tears.

Before you begin using a homeopathic medicine for respiratory allergies, check with a qualified practitioner, and use these treatments under his or her guidance (as well as the advice of your pediatrician), particularly with very young children. Generally, you will be provided with information concerning the standard dosage from the practitioner, or the standard dosage will be indicated on the container. If taking a dose of the medicine causes the child's symptoms to improve, wait until the symptoms return before giving any more to the child. If the children's symptoms do not improve after four hours, administer another dose and wait an additional four hours. Administer homeopathic medicine no more than three times a day, and for no more than a week.

Also administer healthy doses of common sense. Avoid known allergens as much as possible. Give your child plenty of water to keep his or her system flushed of the allergens that can accumulate. Using a humidifier can also help to relieve swollen air passages.

Skin Allergies   Homeopathic medicine offers a range of remedies for allergies related to the skin. Diagnosis of these ailments is focused on the appearance of the skin irritation, associated bodily sensations like sensitivity to heat, and also how they actually occurred in the first place. In treating skin allergies, homeopathic medicine offers remedies that can be taken internally as well as applied to the skin. Homeopaths discourage the use of hydrocortisone, a commonly used over-the-counter remedy, because they view it as an overly potent drug that is absorbed into the circulation system and can lead to hormonal imbalances. Likewise, the use of calamine lotion is discouraged because it masks symptoms. As in other ailments, skin symptoms need to be fully expressed so that the underlying imbalance can be resolved.

Homeopaths often advise their patients to try to figure out what caused the allergic reaction and to avoid it for a week or two, to see if the symptoms clear up on their own. However, the underlying causes of the symptoms can also be treated, especially if they are severe enough to interfere with the child's sleep and other activities. One of the most widely used remedies for skin allergies is Rhus toxicodendron, derived from poison ivy. Its use is indicated for contact dermatitis, with burning, itching, and fluid-filled skin eruptions that seem to be worse at night and in open air. Feelings of restlessness and irritability are also clues that Rhus toxicodendron might be a good match with this set of symptoms.

An allergic reaction in which the skin is inflamed and blistered, but not itching, might call for croton oil derived from Croton tiglium. A child with a rash requiring croton oil might first be able to relieve the itching through scratching it a bit. However, this action causes the rash to become so inflamed that even touching it lightly causes pain.

Other homeopathic remedies are also useful in treating contact dermatitis, with each prescription based on differences in the appearance and associated symptoms of this ailment. Bryonia, for example, is prescribed for a rash that includes dry bumps accompanied by feelings of irritability. Anacardium is used when symptoms include blisters filled with a yellow fluid.

The homeopathic treatment of hives also varies based on the appearance of the hives, how they came about, and whether the symptoms change due to exposure to conditions like heat and cold. The most commonly used medicine for treating hives is Apis, derived from bee venom. Apis is effective on hives that are extremely itchy, and made worse by exposure to warmth, through exercise, for example, or due to a change in the weather. While Apis is used most often, Urtica urens, from stinging nettle, may also be helpful.

Eczema, which often accompanies respiratory symptoms, is commonly treated with medicines aimed at curing the respiratory problems. Homeopaths might treat eczema with sabadilla, for example, arsenicum, or Wyethia, discussed earlier, depending on the specific range of respiratory symptoms associated with the eczema.

Skin allergies are difficult for the layman to treat because the selection of homeopathic medicine is based on subtle differences between groups of related symptoms. For example, it is difficult for a layman to distinguish between various types of blisters or bumps. Thus, it is best to work under the guidance of a qualified practitioner.

Food Allergies What appears to be a food allergy, according to homeopathy, may be the result of toxins that have accumulated in the digestive system and created an imbalance. Treatment is aimed at matching symptoms such as vomiting, nausea, and diarrhea with a homeopathic medicine that mimics these symptoms, and helps the body to bring itself back into balance. Additionally, homeopathic remedies can be helpful in replacing the bodily fluids that are depleted by conditions like vomiting, thus creating an environment for healing to take place.

For children, homeopathic remedies are often a reliable alternative to chemical-based medications that not only add toxins to the system but mask symptoms that will return once the drug wears off, and interfere with natural digestive and healing processes. Many over-the-counter remedies are developed for adults and are really too strong for use in children.

It is also important to keep in mind that a homeopathic physician will sometimes recommend letting food allergy symptoms take their course without any specific intervention. For example, keeping your child away from specific foods that cause allergic reactions, treating diarrhea-induced fluid loss with water to replace the lost fluids, and keeping him or her warm and comfortable until the symptoms have passed might be all that is necessary. Also, because children's digestive systems are still developing, they vomit more easily than adults anyway. This is especially true of babies, in whom the valve that closes off the bottom of the esophagus is not yet fully developed, resulting in a tendency to spit up easily. Vomiting is not necessarily an emergency situation unless it becomes frequent and results in weight loss and dehydration.

Vomiting and diarrhea, even when you suspect they are related to a food allergy, should first be treated without medicine. The lining of the stomach is most likely inflamed, perhaps as a result of the allergy, and food and liquid can irritate it further. First, consult your pediatrician. It is generally recommended that the child be given a minimal amount of liquids for a few hours, maybe for up to six hours, and the symptoms be allowed to calm down. Then begin to replace the fluids with tiny amounts of clear liquids, such as vegetable broth, juice, or flat soda. Avoid milk and animal products.

Over the next day or two, gradually increase the liquids and begin to introduce solid foods like toast and yogurt. Caution: You should not withhold fluids from babies and very young children, but continue to give them small amounts, even a teaspoon at a time. Children are much more susceptible to dehydration because they have a faster metabolism and because their kidneys are still developing. Keep a close eye on children when they are experiencing these symptoms, and be ready to contact a physician if they persist more than a day or two.

Symptoms of dehydration, for adults and children, include a dry mouth, and no tears in the eyes. As dehydration continues, the symptoms include sunken eyes, loss of skin elasticity, and a sunken soft spot on the head in very young children. If you see any of these signs, get your child to a physician, or an emergency room, immediately.

Food allergies in children can also result in abdominal pain. This can be treated with rest and small meals of mild food and clear liquids. This will let the symptoms work themselves out. Also treat the child for related symptoms such as vomiting. Abdominal pain can also result from appendicitis, rather than a food allergy, and when these pains occur without other symptoms, and either continue or worsen, medical attention may be necessary.

Symptoms like abdominal pain, vomiting, and diarrhea, can also be treated with homeopathic medicines, generally given once per hour until the symptoms begin to subside. Medicines should be given every twelve hours if symptoms are less severe. When using a homeopathic medicine for possible food allergy symptoms, you should notice improvements rather quickly. If not, switch to another homeopathic medicine. And again, if symptoms become severe, get medical assistance.

Arsenicum album is one of the more commonly used homeopathic medicines for treating ailments of the gastrointestinal system. Symptoms include vomiting, diarrhea, and stomach or intestinal pain. Other symptoms that point to the need for arsenicum include fearfulness, exhaustion, and restlessness, as well as extreme thirst and chilliness. These symptoms are worse at night, and eating and drinking quickly result in vomiting.

If the major symptom is nausea, with or without diarrhea or vomiting, then ipecac is another homeopathic medicine to consider. A child needing ipecac is most likely not as seriously ill as one needing arsenicum. Colocynth, derived from bitter cucumber, is indicated if the major symptom is abdominal cramps made worse by eating or drinking. This type of cramps can be relieved through gentle pressure on the abdomen, and warmth. Belladonna may also be useful in the early stages of gastrointestinal distress, if the symptoms have come on suddenly.

The homeopathic remedies discussed above are only a selection of those that can be helpful in relieving the symptoms of food allergy. Again, the causes and symptoms of food allergy are unique to the individual, and in most cases cannot be traced to only one source. Homeopathic medicines can contribute to relieving the symptoms as well as helping to provide balance to the system and relieve it of toxins. However, the actual homeopathic "cure" for food allergy includes a healthy dose of avoidance—if a food is known to cause a reaction, your child should be guided in learning to avoid it.

Also keep in mind that it is possible that some of the homeopathic medicines you choose may elicit allergic reactions, even though they are derived from natural substances.

Working with a Homeopathic Physician One of the difficulties in making your own diagnosis of your child's allergies, and in turn choosing a homeopathic medicine, is that you are at best making an educated guess. Your child may be able to report exactly how he or she is feeling, but in most cases, you have to rely on your own observations. While you can discontinue a medicine if it does not seem to be helping, you may waste time and money on medicines that are not working.

A homeopathic physician can help you to avoid these mistakes. He or she will begin by carefully examining your child, while asking you and your child a detailed list of questions about how and when the symptoms occur, and the conditions surrounding these situations. You will be called on to provide detailed information about your child's likes and dislikes, emotional makeup, mental state, and history of childhood illnesses. You may want to bring the baby book along. Also, keep a journal of how your child has behaved in the days before and after an allergy attack, including food eaten, hours of sleep, and the specific symptoms. This information will all be used by the homeopathic practitioner in choosing an initial course of treatment.

As discussed above, a wide range of homeopathic remedies can be helpful in treating childhood allergies, since allergic reactions are symptoms of underlying imbalances. You will need to be a treatment partner with your practitioner. Watch how your child reacts to the medicine and report any changes or improvements in his or her condition. If the symptoms worsen, or other symptoms occur, make sure you let your practitioner know immediately.

If your homeopathic practitioner is not also a qualified medical doctor, let your regular physician know that your child is undergoing homeopathic treatment. Your physician needs to be aware of this to avoid prescribing medications that may interfere with the homeopathic approach. And in the event of any kind of medical emergency, contact your physician to provide emergency treatment and arrange for hospitalization if needed. Many physicians now accept the validity of natural approaches and will work with you and your homeopathic practitioner.

Naturopathy

Naturopaths view allergic rhinitis, hay fever, and other allergies in children as outgrowths of illness and allergic responses that begin during infancy. These allergies begin in the digestive system or gut. Naturopaths stress the importance of breast-feeding infants during the first six months of life, because their digestive systems are not ready for the chemicals and preservatives that they are fed through cow's milk and formula; they have very little protection against them. Their guts are not yet developed, and so their digestive tract is thrown off by these artificial ingredients. The same situation occurs if infants are weaned too early and fed solid foods that also introduce food allergens into their systems. These ingredients are treated by the body as if they were foreign substances, and allergic reactions develop.

With the development of these infant food allergies comes a greater susceptibility to childhood illnesses. Ear infections, for example, can be the result of allergic symptoms that have settled in the ear. Infections are often treated with antibiotics, which add to the problem. Antibiotics further throw the digestive tract off balance by interfering with the natural processes of breaking down and eliminating food, and the allergies worsen. Eczema, allergic rhinitis, hay fever, and asthma often follow, all resulting from what, in children, are essentially food allergies.

Naturopathic practitioners view allergy as a trigger for

asthma, and the treatments are similar for both. The naturopathic approach to juvenile allergy will be discussed here, and asthma treatments will be discussed in more depth in Chapter 7.

Naturopaths treat the causes of all childhood allergies, including allergic rhinitis, hay fever, and skin allergies, with food allergy as the underlying cause. For example, naturopaths believe hay fever is related to food allergies that result in symptoms such as sneezing and congestion. Symptoms can be immediate, and possibly related to sensitivities to foods such as fish, eggs, nuts, or shellfish; or the symptoms can be delayed, and more likely the result of allergies to foods like wheat, chocolate, milk products, or food coloring. Having a low stomach acidity is another factor recognized by naturopaths in the development of allergic reactions, with food staying in the stomach longer and creating imbalances that lead to allergic reactions. Stress is another factor, especially with reactions like eczema.

Food allergy and low stomach acid are also associated with asthma, as is exposure to food additives, like artificial dyes and preservatives. This is discussed in Chapter 7.

Treating Your Child with Naturopathy The primary approach to treating juvenile allergy is through diet, as well as through nutritional supplements and vitamins, and herbal medicines. For children, this begins with an elimination diet, consisting of foods that include chicken, lamb, potatoes, bananas, rice, apples, and vegetables such as broccoli and cabbage. These foods are not likely to result in allergic reactions, and will provide nourishment while the toxins caused by other foods are gradually eliminated from the system. A child normally stays on this diet for a week or more, at which point additional foods can be introduced, one every day or two. The child can be observed for any reactions to these foods. If allergic symptoms occur, the new food should be withdrawn. This requires careful record keeping, but it is an excellent way of designing a diet that works for your child.

Below, naturopathic treatments for the main types of juvenile allergies are described.

Eczema   Eczema in children, as already discussed, is often related to food allergies. Thus, a first defense prescribed by the naturopath would be to use the elimination diet to discover the cause of the eczema, and then eliminate it from the child's diet. Milk products are one of the most common eczema-causing foods, and this might be one of the first foods to be avoided.

Nutritional supplements are also used in treating eczema. For example, children with eczema often have a deficiency in essential fatty acids, which results in a decrease in the ability to fight off inflammation, so evening primrose might be given to balance this deficiency and relieve symptoms. Eating more fish or using a fish oil supplement might also be recommended for their antiallergy and antiinflammatory effects, as would taking bioflavonoids. Vitamin A helps to enhance the overall healthiness of the skin.

Eczema is also treated with botanical medicines. Vaccinium myrtillus, from blueberry leaf, and Prunus spinosa, from blackthorn, are used to inhibit the production of histamines and serve as antiinflammatories. Burdock root has a direct healing effect on eczema by correcting defects in the immune systems of eczema sufferers. Licorice and chamomile can be used in preparations that offer the same temporary relief as cortisone.

Naturopaths believe that cortisone has long-term negative effects on the body. Using cortisone on eczema continues the cascade effect that begins with antibiotics.

Whereas antibiotics for ailments like ear infections may interfere with the digestive system and ultimately result in the histamines being sent to the skin, cortisone sends the histamines on to the lungs, where the result can be allergic rhinitis and asthma.

Naturopaths also recommend the use of a nonoily zinc ointment to relieve the itching associated with eczema, and that only mild soaps be used.

Allergic Rhinitis and Hay Fever Naturopathic treatment for children with allergic rhinitis and hay fever begins with diet. While the elimination diet includes meat, your naturopath may recommend a vegetarian diet for your child, avoiding all meat, fish, dairy products, and eggs. Drinking water is limited to spring water, with avoidance of soda and other stimulants, as well as sugar and salt. The naturopath's allergy diet includes unlimited amounts of vegetables, including lettuce, broccoli, celery, beets, cucumber, and most beans except soy and green beans. Restricted amounts of potatoes are allowed, with most fruits except apples and citrus fruits, and very restricted amounts of grains.

Animal products can cause childhood allergy symptoms. The vegetarian diet alters the metabolism, lowering the tendency toward nasal and lung inflammation. Another benefit is the elimination of any allergens that are being consumed through food, resulting in a gradual detoxification. It's important to work with your child in changing his or her diet. Forcing a child to adopt a diet that is viewed as unexciting, and radically different from that of the other children at school, can cause him or her to feel like an outsider and result in even more stress.

Botanical medicines are also used in treating allergic rhinitis and hay fever. Ephedra is a natural remedy that has been used for thousands of years in treating allergy symptoms. The Ephedra plant contains components that act as antiinflammatory and antiallergy agents. The usefulness of Ephedra diminishes if it is used repeatedly over time, and it is often supplemented by other herbs, like licorice, as well as vitamin C, vitamin B_6, and other nutritional supplements.

Skullcap is another botanical medicine often used by naturopaths in treating allergic rhinitis and hay fever. It has an antiinflammatory action, and inhibits allergy symptoms by combatting the effects of the histamines. Angelica, licorice, onions, and garlic are also among the herbal medicines that a naturopath will draw upon in treating allergy.

Food Allergy   As discussed earlier in this section, naturopaths view most allergies as having their roots in food allergy. Treatment often begins with the elimination diet. This works especially well with specific food allergies because the time between when a food first enters the system and subsequently leads to an allergic reaction is often relatively short. As a result, discovering your child's food allergies may be a relatively simple process.

Naturopaths also recommend the rotary diversified diet for food allergies. This diet helps to keep your child's food allergy symptoms to a minimum by both minimizing exposure to the known allergies as well as preventing new ones. Naturopaths believe that if tolerated foods are eaten on a regular basis, new allergies will not be induced. In the rotary diversified diet, the foods that are tolerated are eaten at specific intervals, every four to seven days. With this routine firmly established, foods that have been known to cause allergic symptoms can gradually be introduced. This way, your child can begin to again enjoy foods that were previously forbidden.

Because of the possibility of reactions caused by eating

foods from the same group, this diet requires some rotation of food groups. This can become a bit complicated until you develop a pattern. Naturopaths who do not specialize in nutrition may bring in another practitioner to help in developing a diet.

Food allergy is often associated with immune system dysfunction. Naturopaths often prescribe nutritional supplements that strengthen the immune system, including selenium, zinc, and B complex. Vitamin C may be recommended as an antihistamine.

Working with Your Naturopath Children are sensitive creatures, and naturopaths avoid harsh medications that might interfere with a child's natural development process. Paying closer attention to what your child eats—avoiding sugar, bleached flour, and preservatives, and choosing food from the major food groups—can have pronounced benefits for your child's health. Vitamin supplements can enhance vitality, and herbal preparations, especially those used in lotions, can be a good substitute for over-the-counter preparations.

However, if your child is in a treatment program with a medical doctor, use caution in making any changes without first talking it over with your doctor. Sudden changes in diet, as discussed earlier, can be stressful. And if your child's allergy symptoms become severe or life threatening you will need to have access to medical help.

Talk with your medical doctor about your naturopath's plan for treating your child's allergies. If he or she is currently receiving desensitization injections or taking antihistamines these treatments may not be compatible with some of the herbal remedies that may be recommended by your naturopath. Discuss the implications with both individuals, particularly potential emergency situations that can result from allergy symptoms. You may be able to use both approaches in tandem, or you may have to make a choice.

Nutrition

Children's foods need to be chosen carefully. Those with food allergies are even more susceptible to excessive use of spices, sugar, and preservatives. Nutritionists treat childhood allergies with a balanced diet that includes avoidance of allergy-triggering foods.

Some food allergies are especially common in children. For example, allergy to cow's milk is fairly common during the first two years of life, and this is treated by avoiding milk and replacing it with soy milk and other substitutes. Allergy to certain grains can also develop in children, and this is also treated by avoiding products that contain wheat, oats, or corn.

If your child has a food allergy, chances are you are aware of it. However, you may need to do some of your own detective work to understand the full range of your child's allergies. When you opt to control your child's food allergies with a nutritional approach, you'll need to work closely with your nutritionist. This work will begin with a food diary in which you'll be asked to record everything that goes into your child's mouth, from food to toothpaste. This diary must be kept night and day, with times and amounts, for one week or more. Your nutritionist will then work with you to find patterns—foods, times of day, and specific symptoms—that point to allergic reaction.

The next step in treating your child's food allergies will be through an elimination diet, with the foods under suspicion placed on a forbidden list, and replaced by a balanced diet that substitutes foods that your child is more likely to tolerate. Your work does not stop here. You'll need to start keeping your food diary again, this time for a week or two, in order to follow your child's progress on the new diet. This will mean recording all foods, amounts, and times of day, as well as any new symptoms that may appear. If the diet is working, the symptoms should subside or disappear.

Elimination is followed by reintroduction. Your child may be presented with tiny amounts of the foods that are suspected to cause allergic reactions, one at a time. This might mean a small bit of chocolate, or a few nuts, or a tiny glass of milk. If he or she has another reaction, then you can be sure that this food needs to go on the forbidden list, at least for the foreseeable future.

Keep in mind that if your child has a reaction to a specific food, he or she is most likely also allergic to the foods in that same family. Additionally, some foods can work together to cause new allergic reactions, and you may not discover this until you combine them quite by accident. Your nutritionist can help you manage these possibilities by providing you with a chart that lists the various food groups to make sure you are avoiding all the foods you need to. He or she can also give you advice as to what foods may combine to cause additional symptoms.

Be prepared to make substitutions when you cook. If your child has an egg allergy, for example, you'll need to know how to substitute for eggs in your cooking. The same goes for wheat, which can often be replaced with oats or barley. A corn allergy may require not only substituting for the corn in a recipe but also watching for the presence of cornstarch in foods like baking powder.

Children are also susceptible to food additives like coloring and preservatives; these artificial chemicals may not only result in allergic reactions but also chronic conditions like hyperactivity and asthma. A dye called tartrazine, referred to as Yellow Number 5, can cause breathing difficulties and headaches in children. Monosodium glutamate can cause chest pains and breathing difficulty. Sulfites, which are often used as a preservative in prepared foods, some seafoods, and in salad bars, can also cause asthma. Your nutritionist can help you to know what food additives to watch out for, and how to read food labels so that you avoid them.

Work closely with your child as you make changes in his or her diet. Sudden changes in diet can be uncomfortable for an adult but traumatic for children. They can result in eating disorders that can be as devastating as the allergies themselves. And when children are forced to eat food that is different from what the other children at school are eating, this sets them apart and can result in damaged self-esteem. Let your child have some control over his diet and make decisions together about what substitutes to choose.

Medical doctors often look to nutrition as a primary treatment for childhood food allergies. He or she may understand enough about nutrition to supervise your child's diet and provide specific recommendations. Increasingly, however, physicians work with nutritionists on diet management, recognizing that designing the right diet is a complicated process requiring the specialized training and experience of a nutritionist. Ask your physician to recommend a nutritionist, if possible, and in any case make sure that he or she is aware that you are seeking the advice of a nutritionist. And have your nutritionist check your child's diet periodically to make adjustments as his or her condition changes.

As always, keep your emergency medical treatment channels open. Some food allergies can be life threatening, including sensitivity to shellfish, nuts, and sulfites, and the span of time between the initial reaction and a life-threatening condition is short.

Psychotherapy

The role that the emotions play in juvenile allergy was discussed earlier in this chapter. Allergic children often don't feel good about themselves. Their symptoms set them apart from siblings and classmates, and their self-esteem suffers. Other children may laugh at the dark circles around their eyes, for example, or the way they constantly sniffle or wipe their noses. Children often don't know how to articulate the way they are feeling, and also may not want to confide in their parents for fear of being viewed as a failure.

A psychotherapist who has expertise in working with children will help your child explore feelings about being allergic, how your child feels around other people, and how allergy symptoms are affecting peer-group acceptance and self-esteem. Allergic children sometimes use their allergies as a coping mechanism, as a means of "getting back at" parents or others who have made them angry, or as a means of gaining attention. Your child's therapist will not only be a good sounding board but will also teach ways of dealing with emotions, and getting needs met, without having to get sick.

Find a psychotherapist who is experienced in working with children with allergies. Weekly sessions may be recommended if your child is having difficulty in coping with day-to-day situations, but this level of intensity may not be needed. The therapist may also recommend a support group with other allergic children. Make sure you choose a therapist with whom you and your child both feel comfortable.

CHAPTER SIX

Adult Asthma

Asthma is a disease of the larger and medium-sized air passages in the lungs, called bronchi. Healthy bronchi are soft and open, with a pink membrane lining. The mucus inside healthy bronchi is kept moving by cilia, which look like little tiny moving hairs. Air moves in and out without noise.

People with asthma have bronchi that are easily irritated. During an asthma attack, the bronchi can go into spasms, and the membranes that line them become swollen and turn red. Also during an asthma attack an excessive amount of mucus is produced. Breathing can become difficult due to the swelling and the extra mucus, with the chest expanding violently to take in air, and the diaphragm pushing it out. This labor results in a breathing noise called wheezing.

Scientists don't really know what causes some people to have asthma, while others are not bothered by it at all. As always, genetics may play a role.

The Symptoms of Asthma

Unlike allergies, with a wide range of symptoms, the symptoms of asthma are simply shortness of breath, wheezing, and to a lesser extent, coughing.

Most asthmatics find the late evening and/or morning

hours to be especially troublesome. This is because asthmatics breathe best when sitting up, so the prone position is not conducive to the easiest breathing. Also, while you sleep, the mucus tends to accumulate, in part because the cilia in the bronchi are not moving as rapidly. You may also find that your wheezing is louder at some times than at others. This is because the loudness depends on where the wheezing is being produced. Wheezing that can barely be heard is being produced in the smaller air passages, while loud wheezing is being produced in the larger upper air passages.

Other symptoms of asthma include drawing in the muscles around the neck and ribs. This drawing in is a result of struggling to breathe in air. Breathing difficulty can also result in bluish lips and drowsiness. These symptoms indicate more severe asthma.

You can start to prevent asthma by keeping track of conditions that bring it on and, as much as possible, trying to avoid them. This is particularly true if your asthma is caused by allergens, such as animal dander.

What Happens During an Attack?

When an individual experiences asthma symptoms, this is generally referred to as an asthma attack. While it is often assumed that asthmatics have difficulty taking in oxygen, people with asthma don't have as much trouble breathing in as they do breathing out.

During normal breathing, air moves from the nose or mouth, through the trachea, and into the bronchi. You lower the diaphragm and expand the ribs to make the lungs fill with air. This is also true for asthmatics. Breathing out is a lot more passive. When you stop breathing in, you automatically breath out.

Here is where the trouble begins for asthmatics.

Breathing out is not so automatic when asthma symptoms are present. If you have asthma, the minute you relax your ribs and let the diaphragm slide up, the obstructed airways block the airflow. The air can't get out. As a result, dead air is trapped in the lungs and you end up breathing at the top of your lungs. This difficulty in exhaling is caused by three factors: secretion of excess mucus, swelling in the airway, and muscle spasm.

For asthmatics, the most noticeable symptom is wheezing.

What Happens Inside During an Attack

The airway through which the oxygen passes during breathing is normally clear. It is lined with ciliated cells, which look like little tiny hairs that keep the mucus moving. Underneath the cilia is a membrane and below that, muscle. Again, this is during normal breathing.

During a bout with asthma, your airway fills with an excessive amount of sticky mucus as well as with other kinds of debris, including two kinds of white blood cells. Also, some of the cells that should be lining and protecting the airway lift off and clump together in the airway. As a result, the airway now contains unprotected spots that become irritated and sore like skin that has been scraped.

With all of these additional materials in the airways, the membrane underneath the ciliated cells becomes very thick. Additionally, this membrane becomes full of inflamed cells, called eosinophils and neutrophils. The muscle layer thickens and contraction occurs. The mucous glands become enlarged and actively secrete more mucus, which further fills up the airway.

Wheezing, coughing, and shortness of breath—the standard symptoms of an asthma attack—are a result of this constriction and irritation in the airway.

Triggers of an Asthma Attack

A range of factors can cause an asthma attack. Some factors are allergic rhinitis, stress, and environmental pollution. These factors are described below.

Allergy   Not all individuals who suffer from allergies also have asthma, and not all asthma sufferers have allergies. However, allergy is the factor most likely to trigger an asthma attack, particularly in children (this will be further explored in Chapter 7). In fact, 90 percent of children with asthma also have allergies. For those under thirty with asthma, 70 percent are allergic. Approximately 50 percent of those over thirty with asthma also have allergies. Allergens that are inhaled, such as dust, mold, dander, and pollen, are especially likely to lead to an asthma attack. To a lesser extent, food allergies can also trigger an asthma attack, though this is rare. Additionally, many asthmatics also experienced eczema as children.

What happens during an allergic reaction was described in Chapter 4. Mast cells are heavily concentrated in the mucous membranes. These cells contain many IgE antibodies, which are proteins manufactured by the body as protection from bacteria and viruses. In allergic people, these antibodies are also directed against harmless substances like pollen and dust. Histamine is released, which leads to an allergic reaction. Histamine can interact with the airways and produce the changes that result in asthma.

Because hay fever is a seasonal ailment, if your asthma is triggered by hay fever your asthma problems will also be seasonal. Breathing difficulties resulting from hay fever will more likely occur in the late evening, when waking up in the morning, or after being outside. Once the season is over, chances are the incidence of asthma will also diminish. Asthma that results from allergies to animals, house dust, or smoke is harder to control. Attacks triggered by these allergens can occur at any time, especially when the concentration of allergens is highest. Thus, attacks can occur during the middle of the night, if you are closed up in the house with a pet.

Allergy is not always a trigger for asthma, but it can be if one of the following factors is present:

- The asthma began during childhood
- The asthma symptoms occur in the fall or spring, or become worse during these seasons
- Other allergic symptoms also occur, including runny nose, hay fever, or eczema
- A relative, such as a parent, sibling, aunt, or uncle, also has allergies

If allergens are an asthma trigger for you, the ones you need to watch out for are pollen, mold, animal dander, house dust, and cockroach droppings.

Infection   Respiratory infections are another common trigger for asthma. Viral infections produce an added irritation in the throat, lungs, and sinuses. A cold may worsen and turn into an infection of the lungs, causing coughing and wheezing. Sinuses may also drain mucus down into the lower respiratory tract.

Activity   Strenuous activity, particularly exercise, is also a major trigger for asthma. Individuals vary in terms of their ability to tolerate activity; some with a history of asthma can exercise long and hard and remain symptomless, while others may start wheezing after a few minutes of exertion. Up to 85 percent of allergic asthmatics experience wheezing during or after exercise. Yet it is not uncommon for some asthmatics to have no history of allergies, and to experience symptoms like wheezing and coughing only after exercise. Other symptoms of exercise-related asthma include accelerated heart rate, coughing, and chest tightness.

Here are the exercises that tend to cause wheezing:

• Running on a track or outside
• Treadmill running
• Bicycling
• Aerobics

Swimming is the exercise that tends to be best for asthmatics. It is available year-round in a warm and humid atmosphere. The horizontal swimming position helps move mucus from the bottom of the lung. And swimming keeps the upper body muscles toned. Other sports that require only short bursts of energy are also recommended, including baseball, football, wrestling, golfing, and gymnastics.

Seasonal differences also affect responses to exercise, with the chances of an asthmatic reaction after exercise higher, for example, during spring pollen season and when the air is cold. Exposure to cold air and low humidity may worsen asthma symptoms because both of these conditions increase heat loss from the airways. And exercising in air that has not been humidified and warmed can result in blocked breathing passages. Cold weather sports like skiing and ice hockey are not recommended for asthmatics because of the combined effects of strenuous exercise with cold air.

Stress and Emotion Your emotional state can have a major effect on asthma, yet as a trigger for an asthma attack emotion is the most difficult to assess. Some practitioners view asthma as being totally the result of emotional states, while others are less convinced of the connection. In either case, it is not uncommon for asthma symptoms to be more severe when stress is also present. It can also be argued that it is possible to have an emotional response to an asthma attack, with feelings such as fear and panic.

Environment   Air quality can also trigger an asthma attack, or at least make an asthma condition worsen. The potential irritants that can trigger asthma include:

- Strong odors and sprays, including perfumes, household cleaners, cooking fumes, paints, and varnishes.

- Air pollutants

- Tobacco smoke

- Chemicals like coal dust, chalk dust, and talcum powder

These substances are often present in school and work environments, and asthma can be worsened by the vapors, dusts, fumes, and gases present in these situations, as well as during the trip to and from home.

Other Chemical Factors   Asthma can also be triggered by chemicals that are ingested. Aspirin, ibuprofin, and other nonsteroid drugs take away pain by interfering with the formation of agents called prostaglandins. An allergy to aspirin can result in a severe asthma attack, and can also be related to sinus problems.

Ingesting sulfites can also trigger asthma. Sulfites are used primarily as a preservative in wine, but are found in some prepared foods. Sulfites are discussed in Chapter 10.

TREATING YOUR ASTHMA WITH NATURAL MEDICINE

Allopathic doctors generally focus their efforts on treating the symptoms of asthma and, since these symptoms can become life threatening, this focus is your first line of defense. If your asthma symptoms are also triggered by allergic rhinitis, your medical doctor may be treating you with desensitization injections. Natural medicine takes a more holistic approach to asthma.

The alternative approaches to treating asthma through natural medicine are aimed at relieving symptoms as well as treating underlying causes. Acupressure and acupuncture, for example, help to repair any imbalances that may be causing asthma. Homeopathy helps to eliminate toxins from the body. Relaxation-oriented practices like meditation help relieve the stress that can contribute to asthma.

Keep the difference between healing your condition and treating your symptoms in mind as you make decisions about what natural medicine alternatives you may want to try for yourself. Always discuss any treatment plans with your treating physician to make sure they are appropriate for you.

Acupressure

Acupressure has been demonstrated to be highly successful in helping individuals with asthma to breathe better by focusing on relaxing the muscles in the bronchi. Acupressure is described in more depth in Chapter 3.

An acupressure practitioner will use a wide range of techniques to treat asthma, focusing on strengthening your natural defenses as well as relieving symptoms. Here are some exercises that you can try at home:

Wheezing and Coughing   Wheezing and coughing can be relieved by pressing just below the upper tip of the shoulder blade, near the spine. Reach over your shoulder with your right hand to locate the point between the tip of your shoulder blade and your spine. Press into this area with your fingertips while taking long and deep breaths. Then use your other arm to repeat the exercise on the other side of your spine.

Breathing Difficulties and Congestion   Breathing difficulties and chest congestion are relieved by using an acupressure point below the collarbone. Press into the indentations directly below your collarbone with your thumbs. Gradually apply pressure on both sides while breathing deeply and slowly. Continue this for five breaths.

Coughing   To relieve the coughing associated with asthma, begin by pressing the indentation of the wrist crease, beneath the base of your thumb, with the thumb of the other hand. Take a few deep breaths while maintaining pressure, then press into the center of the base of the thumb with your index finger of the other hand. Take a few more deep breaths while pressing. Now make a fist with your other hand and stimulate these two points by rubbing your fist into the hand. Continue this action for up to a minute, then repeat the exercise beginning with the other hand.

Tension and Emotional Stress   To relieve the tension and emotional stress that can contribute to asthma symptoms, begin by making fists in front of your chest with the thumbs pointing up. Place your thumbs on the outer area of the chest and press on the muscles that run horizontally under the collarbone. Locate the sensitive spot on the chest muscles and press into that point with your thumbs. As you press, relax your neck, allowing your head to hang forward into your chest. Relax into this position as you continue pressing the acupressure points, and breathe deeply for a minute or more.

As discussed in Chapter 4, working with a qualified acupressure practitioner can help you to gain increased benefits.

Acupuncture

The philosophy of acupuncture, and its use as a treatment, is described in Chapters 2 and 3. Acupuncturists view asthma as the result of an imbalance of *chi*. In a state of good health, *chi* should flow evenly throughout the organs of the body. Blockages in this flow can lead to imbalances that result in illness. This imbalance can be caused by a range of factors, including a diet laden with animal fat and food additives, stress, and lack of exercise.

Asthma is viewed primarily as an overabundance of water going to the lung area. The lungs are not only involved in breathing, but also help to protect the rest of the body from factors such as damp air. In asthmatics this deficiency in lung energy is the result of a deficiency in the kidney yang, resulting in feelings of fear that are carefully hidden behind an overcalm exterior. This may explain the strong emotions that often accompany asthma symptoms. This combination of deficient kidney yang and excess water in the lungs is diagnosed by examining the tongue and pulse. The tongue is often coated by a pale, whitish moss, and the pulse is intermittent.

Treatment for this condition will begin with eliminating the blockages to the kidneys to rebalance the yin and yang in this organ. Once the kidneys are back in balance, the oversupply of liquid that is in effect backing up into the lungs should also begin to fall back into balance. The asthma symptoms should clear up.

Acupuncture treatment is not an overnight process, though you may begin to experience some relief rather quickly. Most likely, you will need to visit your practitioner on a regular basis to allow treatment to undo what might be the result of years of accumulated damage to your system. As always, you should let your medical doctor know that you have decided to undergo acupuncture treatment. You will still need to have medication and treatment available to you in case of an emergency.

Affirmations

Affirmations are helpful both in reducing stress as well as promoting an attitude of healing. The use of affirmations is described in more depth in Chapter 3.

Here are a few affirmations to use for asthma:

- My lungs are strong and healthy. I can breathe deeply and freely.
- The universe is providing me with the ability to breathe abundantly.
- My lungs are free of congestion.

Say your affirmations in the morning, when your mind is free, and at night before you go to sleep. You may also want to write your affirmations on paper, and put them up in your bedroom and in the bathroom, to remind yourself to think positive thoughts.

Aromatherapy

The use of natural inhalants in treating asthma symptoms has a long history and early treatment of asthma included inhaling scent extracted from plants such as eucalyptus. Thus, many of the essential oils used in aromatherapy can be helpful in treating adult asthma. As with many other natural treatments, aromatherapy can alleviate some of the symptoms of asthma as well as strengthen the body's natural defenses. Aromatherapy is discussed in Chapter 3.

As with other ailments, certain aromas affect subconscious parts of your brain that cause a release of positive energy that counteracts the asthma symptoms. Because asthma involves the lungs, breathing essential oils can help clear the lungs of congestion, which makes breathing easier and reduces wheezing. Other oils have a calming effect that alleviates the sense of fear and panic that often accompanies asthma.

The best place to begin to draw upon the wisdom of aromatherapy is with a qualified aromatherapist. This individual will listen as you discuss your symptoms and what stimuli bring on an asthma attack. The aromatherapist will also ask you questions about your household and your normal routine. He or she will then make recommendations about the essential oils that might be most helpful, and how and when to use them. Because asthma involves the lungs, the aroma lamp will be a standard part of your treatment. Additionally, hot compresses, when placed directly over the lungs, can also be useful in clearing congestion.

A range of essential oils is useful in relieving the symptoms of asthma, including congestion, difficulty in breathing, coughing, and wheezing. A few of these essential oils are discussed below.

Lemon Balm   Lemon balm oil is extracted from the herb, Melissa officinalis, which for centuries has been associated with treating anxiety, tension, circulation, and heart disturbances, as well as asthma. To use lemon balm oil in treating asthma symptoms, place a few drops in an aroma lamp. Lemon balm has a pleasing aroma that will permeate your home. Keep in mind that the best way to obtain real lemon balm oil is through an aromatherapist, and it is expensive. Otherwise, what you buy may be produced from a plant such as lemongrass. Also keep in mind that lemon balm should not be taken internally.

Cedar   The essential oil of the cedar tree, particularly those grown in Morocco and Algeria, offers lifegiving and calming effects. Cedar oil also has beneficial effects on the bronchial system and is a good expectorant that helps to relieve coughing. For asthma, place a few drops of cedar oil in an aroma lamp. If desired, cedar can be mixed with lemon or hyssop oils.

Cypress   The oil of the cypress tree acts in harmony with the central nervous system, bringing serenity and strengthening connective tissues. Cypress is an old remedy for coughing, including the convulsive coughs associated with asthma. It is known to stop excess flows and as such is an excellent expectorant that relieves lung congestion. Place a few drops of cypress oil in an aroma lamp, or obtain a salve from your aromatherapist that includes cypress oil and rub it directly on the back and chest.

Eucalyptus   The healing powers of eucalyptus have been, and continue to be, widely known as a treatment for respiratory difficulties. In fact, many cough medications available in your drugstore contain eucalyptus, as do various topical preparations for treating pain. The whole breathing process is actually aided by eucalyptus, because it both helps to regenerate lung tissue as well as acting as an expectorant and decongestant. Place a few drops of eucalyptus in an aroma lamp for relief of coughing and wheezing. You may also want to talk to your aromatherapist about obtaining a natural ointment that you can rub into your chest at night.

Rosemary Of all the essential oils used in the practice of aromatherapy, rosemary is among the most common. Rosemary is believed to strengthen and promote awareness because of its effect on the central nervous system. As such, it is especially useful in conjunction with meditation and visualization. For treating general asthma symptoms, place a few drops of rosemary essential oil in an aroma lamp. Rosemary may also be taken internally but, as always, check with an aromatherapist first.

Aromatherapy can be useful in conjunction with meditation and yoga by helping to create a calming and health-promoting environment. Keep in mind that your asthma can react negatively to certain aromas, and if you begin to experience asthma symptoms as a result of using an essential oil, remove it from your presence immediately. Additionally, if symptoms persist, get into contact with a physician. Do this immediately if breathing becomes difficult.

Botanical Medicine

Some of the earliest treatments available for asthma were based on botanical medicine, with herbal preparations used in treating wheezing, coughing, restricted breathing, and overproduction of mucus. The botanical medicine approach to asthma includes both prevention and treatment of symptoms. The starting place for treatment is through detoxification of the system to rid it of impurities, followed by the treatment of specific symptoms, and then strengthening the weakened areas. Botanical medicine is described in Chapters 2 and 3.

When using herbs to treat your asthma symptoms, some general guidelines should be followed. Most herbs are relatively mild, and should be used in large enough doses to gain the desired results. Following the directions carefully, and consulting with your practitioner, will help you here. Also keep in mind that some herbs can be toxic, and others should not be used if you are pregnant, nursing a child, or have diabetes or other conditions. Not only should you talk to your botanical medicine practitioner about these concerns, but consult with your physician as well before taking any herbal remedy. One single herb can have many properties, meaning that it can have a wide range of positive effects on your body that go beyond relief of asthma symptoms. Some herbs act as expectorants or decongestants, others are antiasthmatic in nature, while still others rejuvenate the respiratory and other systems. Herbs may also be used in combination, with some taken to treat symptoms, and others used for their rejuvenating and strengthening effects. Using herbs in combination is best undertaken with the guidance of a practitioner.

Herbs can be used in a variety of ways when treating asthma. Compresses and oils made with herbs can be placed on your chest for a short period of time or even overnight to help relieve asthma congestion and mucus production. Herbs can also be ingested in teas or consumed in other ways. When consuming herbs, use caution. Make sure you have purchased the herb in a form that allows for consumption, and either read the directions carefully in a botanical medicine book, or work with a practitioner. Also keep in mind that the use of herbs may affect the medical treatment you may be receiving, especially since many medications are derived from herbs. Consult with your physician to make sure he or she is aware of this treatment and supports it.

Here are some of the most commonly used herbs in treating asthma and how you can use them at home:

Ginger Congestion and mucus production can be relieved by using a compress made from ginger. Mix a few drops of a tincture of ginger, which you can purchase from a health food store, with four tablespoons of whole wheat flour and enough water to make a paste. Spread it on a piece of cotton cloth and then lay it on your chest. Leave it on for at least an hour, or even overnight.

Congestion and coughing can also be relieved by using a tea made of fresh gingerroot. Follow these directions for making ginger tea:

1. Grate two inches of gingerroot.
2. Place it in a teapot.
3. Boil one quart of water in a separate container.
4. Pour it over the grated ginger in the teapot.
5. Cover the teapot and let it steep at least fifteen minutes.
6. Drink it warm or cool.

Drink the ginger tea a few times per day, or until the symptoms disappear.

To relieve congestion and dry out excess mucus, try a mixture of the powders of dried ginger, black pepper, and aniseed. Combine small amounts of each of these powders and then mix it with either warm milk or a teaspoon of honey. This mixture is taken internally.

Angelica   Angelica is a bitter herb that, when taken in a warm tea, strengthens the lungs and relieves congestion. To create angelica tea, use one ounce of angelica root for one pint of water, and follow the directions for making ginger tea. Drink one cup three times per day. Angelica can increase the amount of sugar in your blood and should be avoided by diabetics.

Eucalyptus   A small amount of properly diluted eucalyptus oil, rubbed directly into your chest, will help relieve the coughing associated with asthma.

You can also treat coughing with the following recipe: Mix an ounce each of the essential oil of cinnamon, eucalyptus, thyme, camphor, and marjoram. Also add a few drops of olive oil to dilute this mixture. Store this mixture in a bottle. Spread it on your chest at bedtime—it will have a healing and soothing action that will help relieve a hacking cough and associated congestion.

Black Pepper   Black pepper has long been used as an expectorant, for relieving the overproduction of mucus and excessive coughing. Black pepper can be simply taken with food. Or it can be combined with a pinch of aniseed and gingerroot, and combined with honey, to form a relatively pleasant-tasting paste. Mix a teaspoon of the paste with hot water to make a tea, and take up to three times per day.

Coltsfoot   Coltsfoot herb is derived from the leaves and flowers of the coltsfoot plant, and is a bitter herb that has a long history of use in treating cough and in relieving wheezing and labored breathing. Because of its healing nature, it is useful not only for occasional relief of symptoms but also for use on a daily basis to strengthen the respiratory system and prevent asthma attacks. Treat yourself with coltsfoot by making a tea of one ounce of dried coltsfoot herb in a pint of water. Follow the directions for making ginger tea. Drink up to three cups per day when you are experiencing symptoms. You may also want to drink a cup every morning as part of your morning routine, as a preventive measure. Coltsfoot is not recommended for pregnant or nursing women, or for use with young children.

Ginko   Ginko is a bitter-tasting herb derived from the nuts and leaves of the ginko tree. It can be slightly toxic (use under the guidance of a practitioner). Ginko has long been used as an expectorant, and relieves both the coughing and wheezing associated with asthma. Ginko can be ingested in a tea, with one ounce of ginko herb (derived from the leaves of the tree, as opposed to the nuts) in a pint of water, following the same method as that used in making ginger tea. Drink the tea one to three times per day.

Working with Your Botanical Medicine Practitioner   You can experience the benefits of botanical medicine in treating your asthma by trying the remedies described above. There are many good books on the market that illustrate how herbs can be used in treating a range of illnesses. However, if you want to get serious about herbs and experiment with a complete treatment plan, the best place to start is with a practitioner. Botanical medicine practitioners may be difficult to locate depending on where you live. Consult your local health food store, where practitioners may be buying their supplies as well as advertising. Metaphysical churches, community education organizations, and local colleges and universities may also be sources of information.

Your practitioner will recognize asthma symptoms as unique to you—the result of a combination of factors that may include heredity, diet, lifestyle, and the environment you live in. Most likely, he or she will focus on the herbs available in your environment in selecting the best treatment course. And your treatment may include not only herbal remedies for specific symptoms like wheezing but also herbs to remove toxins from your system and to increase your physical stamina. Don't be surprised if you are also asked to make changes in your diet.

Follow your practitioner's guidelines. However, be sure to also consult with your physician as some herbal preparations, especially those that are taken internally, may interact with asthma medications. If the treatments don't seem to help you, or if your symptoms seem to be appearing more often or worsening in severity, let your practitioner know. You'll need to have changes made in your treatment plan.

Botanical medicine can be used with treatments such as acupressure and acupuncture. It is not a good match with aromatherapy or homeopathy because many herbs and essential oils are derived from the same plant, and the two approaches may not work well together.

Breathing Exercises

One way to keep your breathing as strong as possible is through exercises that involve the lungs, diaphragm, and abdominal muscles.

As you breathe in air, the diaphragm moves downward to enlarge the chest cavity, allowing the lungs to fill with air, while the abdominal muscles relax. When you exhale, the diaphragm moves up and squeezes the air out. So, while the chest muscles are important, it's really your diaphragm that is doing a lot of the work.

Good breathing results from your diaphragm working in concert with your abdominal muscles. The following exercises will help you to strengthen your breathing. Before you do any of these exercises, make sure you are wearing comfortable clothes that do not restrict your chest or abdomen, and clear out your nasal passages by blowing your nose.

Exercise 1

1. Sit in an upright position and place your hands over your upper abdomen.
2. Take a deep breath while relaxing your abdominal muscles and allowing your stomach to stick out.
3. Press on your stomach and exhale. Pull in your abdominal muscles so they are as flat as possible.
4. Repeat this exercise up to ten times.

Exercise 2

1. Lie flat on your back, with one hand resting across the middle of your chest and the other hand across your abdomen.
2. Relax your muscles, and then breathe in deeply through your nose. Let your stomach stick out as you fill your lungs.
3. Exhale slowly, pressing on your abdomen inward and upward. Keep pressing on your abdomen until all of the air in your lungs has been exhaled.
4. Repeat this exercise up to ten times.

Exercise 3

1. Lie on your back, legs drawn up, with your arms locked around your legs.
2. Inhale slowly.
3. As you exhale, lift your feet off the floor by pulling your legs toward your chest. Use your arms to help pull.
4. Repeat this exercise up to ten times.

Follow these directions carefully to make sure you do the exercises correctly. And practice them often, even daily, but progress at your own pace. For example, you may want to do only one or two of each the first day, then gradually build up until you can perform ten of each. You may find that the exercises cause you to feel like coughing, or expectorating. If this is a simple cough, don't worry about it. If it is a hard cough, and makes you feel tired, you may want to talk to your physician.

Exercise

If you were an asthmatic child, you probably avoided physical activity in school. Not only did it make your asthma symptoms worse but it probably made you feel bad about yourself if you couldn't keep up with the other kids. But exercise was and still is an important ingredient in keeping you healthy. The benefits of exercise are both physiological and psychological. Regular physical exercise builds up your lungs, strengthens your body, and gives you more energy. Exercise also gives you a greater feeling of control over your life and improves your self-esteem. And it makes you look better.

The basic rule in setting up an exercise program is to

choose an activity that fits within your own specific limitations, but that you also enjoy. If you haven't been exercising, don't start out trying to jog five miles a day, especially if you hate running. Another rule of thumb is to exercise on a regular basis; three times a week is generally recommended. Choose an activity that will get your cardiovascular system stimulated, like swimming or riding a stationary bicycle for a half hour or so. Even a brisk walk can accomplish this. Don't overexert yourself, particularly when you are getting started, and avoid allergens like dust and pollen and excessively cold air that may trigger your asthma.

Before you start an exercise program, talk with your physician and see what he or she recommends for you. Make sure you take any necessary precautions in terms of having medication and emergency assistance available, and follow your physician's guidelines for getting started slowly and building up. Then watch your stamina and your self-esteem start growing.

Holistic Massage

Anxiety, frustration, anger, fear, and other stress-related feelings can accumulate in your system and manifest themselves in physical symptoms. And if you suffer from asthma, these feelings will most likely result in symptoms like congested breathing and wheezing. Holistic massage, with its emphasis on restoring a sense of being relaxed, centered, and in control, can help you to prevent the overload of stress that leads to asthma symptoms, as well as help you to return to a state of relaxation when the symptoms are under way.

Holistic massage is described in Chapter 4, and you may want to review this section. Keep in mind that the parts of your body work together as a whole, and it is important to focus your massage efforts on all parts of the body, from the head to the feet, to promote a state of complete relaxation. Still, as with treating allergic rhinitis and hay fever, pay close attention to relaxing the chest and shoulders because, as a result of breathing difficulties, you may be carrying much of your tension in this area.

While you can schedule a session with a practitioner of holistic massage and receive many of the benefits of this practice, it is best practiced with a partner, like a close friend or loved one. The two of you can use massage to promote mutual understanding and trust that will also enhance your well-being.

Homeopathy

Homeopathic physicians approach the treatment of asthma with extreme caution. When your breathing becomes congested and labored, asthma can turn into a life-threatening condition. For this reason homeopathic practitioners recognize the need for conventional medications, and the ongoing care of a physician, to assure that emergency care is readily available in the event of a serious asthma attack.

With these cautions in mind, homeopathy does offer assistance for asthma sufferers, with remedies that help to strengthen the respiratory system, as well as provide relief for mild wheezing congestion. When asthma-related wheezing is minor, and the breathing is not seriously labored, practitioners first recommend that you drink plenty of liquids. Rapid breathing depletes your body of water, and drinking a lot of water helps to replace these liquids, while also helping to loosen the mucus that is clogging up your breathing passages. Also try some breathing exercises, discussed in a later section in this chapter, to help strengthen your lungs and help you relax.

For ongoing relief, you may also want to try a homeopathic medicine.

Treating Asthma with Homeopathy Because asthma is the result of a range of factors, including genetic predisposition, homeopathy may be limited in some cases as a complete cure. However, even if you are suffering from chronic asthma, you most likely experience periods of time in which you are relatively free of asthma symptoms. If your asthma is allergy related, for example, you may suffer less in the winter. Or maybe you suffer less when you are not under stress. Homeopathy can help you to extend these periods of better health by building up your constitution, as well as offer relief from minor symptoms.

Arsenicum Album The most commonly used homeopathic medicine for asthma is arsenicum. Symptoms that are a match for arsenicum include feelings of fearfulness and restfulness, often related to the panic that many asthmatics experience when they cannot breathe adequately. The asthma symptoms most likely worsen at night, with wheezing and congestion increasing to the point that you toss and turn and constantly get up to take deep breaths. If your asthma condition might benefit from arsenicum you most likely also experience a feeling of weakness. A cough usually accompanies these symptoms, as well as chills, and thirst. If you have these symptoms but they do not noticeably worsen at night, you may still be a candidate for arsenicum.

Pulsatilla Pulsatilla, derived from windflower, is an alternate medicine for asthma. This choice is based not only on asthma symptoms but also behavior. For example, if you feel overly affectionate or tearful and afraid of being left alone, these are pulsatilla symptoms. Asthma-related symptoms indicating a need for pulsatilla include wheezing that either begins, or worsens, during the evening and night. Coughing, accompanied by the need to bring up phlegm that has accumulated in the chest, is another symptom, as is a worsening of symptoms after eating.

Ipecac If the asthma symptoms include a large amount of phlegm in the chest, ipecac is the recommended homeopathic medicine. Symptoms associated with a need for ipecac may include more extreme wheezing, accompanied by a rattling of mucus deep within the chest. The presence of mucus is also obvious during coughing, which can become so intense that it leads to gagging and vomiting. Nausea may also be present. The symptoms associated with a need for ipecac often lead to exhaustion, characterized by a pale and sick appearance.

Spongia Asthma symptoms that do not include phlegm, but instead a dryness, often evidenced by a harsh, dry cough, indicate a need for Spongia, which is derived from roasted sponge. Other symptoms associated with a need for Spongia are noisy and labored breathing with a whistling sound. These symptoms may come after being chilled or having a cold. Wheezing may worsen during sleep, with breathing becoming more labored when lying down. Wheezing may lessen after a warm drink.

If you administer your own homeopathic medicine for asthma, do it carefully and only after consulting with your doctor. The first three doses should be given every two hours, then discontinued as soon as there is some improvement. If there is no improvement after the third dose, wait an hour and try a new medicine, also following it with two additional doses every two hours. If symptoms do not improve, and especially if they worsen, contact a physician immediately. Don't take these medicines more than once in two hours, and don't take more than ten doses in two days.

Working with Your Homeopathic Practitioner   If you are an asthma sufferer, you are probably aware that asthma symptoms can change and worsen quickly. When using a homeopathic medicine, keep in close contact with a practitioner, even on a daily basis when you are in the midst of using a medicine to treat specific symptoms. It's important to keep your practitioner abreast of how the medicines are affecting you, so that changes can be made quickly. As always, if you experience a sudden change in symptoms, including severe shortness of breath or a sore throat with difficulty in swallowing, contact a medical doctor.

Try to work with a homeopathic physician who is also a medical doctor, preferably one who has experience in working with asthma patients. He or she will be most qualified to assess your symptoms and set up a treatment program that provides you not only with relief of your symptoms but helps build up your system to withstand attacks. Remember that homeopathic medicine can help you relieve your symptoms but may not be able to provide you with a total cure.

If your homeopathic physician is not also a medical doctor, you should let your physician know that you are using homeopathic remedies. He or she can still provide you with medicines to use in the event of severe asthma symptoms, and can also serve as the first contact in the case of an emergency. Homeopathy can be supplemented by yoga, exercise, and meditation to help you breathe better and also relax.

Journal Writing

Asthma symptoms are often related to feeling fearful, angry, frustrated, or just pent up. You might find yourself having a range of feelings before or during an attack. Maybe you know exactly what you are feeling and why, or maybe you're not sure. And what do you do with all of these feelings?

Keeping a journal is a way of exploring your thoughts and feelings while also keeping a record of them. You may want to use your journal to explore feelings you are having, where you think they're coming from, and how they're affecting you. If you're enraged at someone and can't confront them directly, you can write a few pages about what you wish you could do about it.

Your journal belongs to you, and as long as you keep it in a safe place, you can write anything in it you want. You can even describe your asthma symptoms and what they feel like, any fears you have, and how you felt before and after. Your journal lets you express your emotions, at least on paper. And you may even start to see some patterns emerge in terms of the feelings you are having just before an attack. What could you do differently? Explore that in a few pages of your journal.

There is no specific way to keep a journal. Simply find a notebook you're comfortable writing in, set some time aside each day to write for a few minutes, and keep it in a safe place. The most important guideline is to loosen up and write what's on your mind, without censoring yourself. That may take some practice, but over time your journal may be one of the first places you go when you need to ventilate. You may want to take a class in journal writing, or buy a book that covers this topic.

Macrobiotics

The primary approach of macrobiotics for treating asthma is through the macrobiotic diet, which is described in Chapter 4. Asthma, especially when caused by allergic rhinitis, is viewed as the result of a buildup of yin, caused by eating excessive amounts of yin foods. These foods include dairy products, especially cold milk, as well as fruit and sugar and food additives. When yin builds up in the system the body becomes so overburdened that it begins to store the excess, rather than eliminating it. The excesses stored by the body include mucus, which causes congestion in the lungs, and symptoms like difficult breathing and wheezing.

Macrobiotic practitioners also associate asthma with excessive liquid, which causes the kidneys to be overworked and unable to eliminate excess liquid and toxins. While the standard macrobiotic diet is recommended for treating asthma, additional recommendations include limiting the amount of fluid by drinking less and not cooking with large amounts of water. Limiting yin foods is also recommended. In addition to the macrobiotic diet, practitioners also use botanical remedies such as placing a hot ginger compress on the chest to relieve congestion.

As always, talk with your medical doctor before you make changes in your diet and in your asthma treatment. Make sure the diet will not interfere with any other conditions you have, like diabetes. And also make sure that medications, and treatment, are available in case of an emergency.

Meditation

Meditation helps you to relieve stress and create a sense of inner peace. When you begin to feel asthma symptoms coming on, with your chest tightening and wheezing, you can use meditation techniques to place yourself in a relaxed state. By being relaxed, you'll be less likely to feel panic, which can result in more chest tightening. To learn the best approach to meditation, refer to Chapter 4.

Naturopathy

Naturopathy views asthma in much the same way as it does allergic rhinitis and hay fever, and there are also many similarities in treatment. Naturopaths look to three major causes in determining the factors that lead to asthma. The first of these is food allergies that result in the symptoms of allergic rhinitis or hay fever. These symptoms can be immediate, and possibly related to allergies to foods such as fish, eggs, nuts, and shellfish; or the symptoms can be delayed, and more likely the result of allergies to foods like wheat, chocolate, milk products, and food coloring. These symptoms in turn serve as a trigger for asthma.

A low stomach acidity is another factor recognized by naturopaths in the development of allergic rhinitis and hay fever, with food staying in the stomach longer and creating imbalances that lead to allergic reactions and then asthma.

Exposure to food additives is also viewed by naturopaths as one of the causes of asthma. Artificial dyes and preservatives like sulfur dioxide, for example, are used in packaged foods and drinks and may trigger asthma.

Treating Asthma with Naturopathy Naturopaths treat asthma primarily through diet. The most highly recommended asthma diet is vegetarian, avoiding all meat, fish, dairy products, and eggs. Drinking water is limited to spring water, though herbal tea is allowed. All coffee, soda, and other stimulants, as well as sugar and salt, must be avoided. This diet does include unlimited amounts of vegetables, including lettuce, broccoli, celery, beets, cucumber and most beans except soy and green beans. Restricted amounts of potatoes are allowed, with most fruits except apples and citrus fruits, and very restricted amounts of grains.

The vegetarian diet should lead to improvement of symptoms after approximately four months, though it may be necessary to stay on it for a year or more. The benefit of this diet is that it eliminates the food allergens, resulting in a gradual detoxification. Nutritional supplements are often used in treating asthma. Vitamin B_6 can help decrease the number of asthma attacks, and cause them to be less severe. Vitamin B_{12} helps prevent asthma symptoms brought on by exposure to sulfites. Vitamin C can have a range of benefits for asthma sufferers. It helps to prevent severe bronchial constriction, and may even help to prevent attacks as well as serve as a possible defense against allergens. Carotenes strengthen the lining of the respiratory tract, while vitamin E is antiinflammatory. Naturopaths vary in their use of supplements and vitamins in treating asthma, however it is not uncommon for a practitioner to prescribe one or more of these as a component of treatment.

Naturopaths will also recommend the use of botanical medicines in treating asthma. These medicines include Ephedra, a natural remedy used for thousands of years in treating allergy symptoms. The Ephedra plant contains components that act as antiinflammatory and antiallergy agents; a synthetic compound made from Ephedra, called ephedrine, is used in many prescription medications for asthma and hay fever. The usefulness of Ephedra diminishes if it is used repeatedly over time, and it is often supplemented by other herbs, like licorice, as well as vitamin C, vitamin B_6, and other nutritional supplements.

Ephedra is often used with herbal expectorants like lico-rice or senega to help clear the respiratory tract of mucus.

The herbal medicine, skullcap, is similar in effect to drugs like aspirin and ibuprofen, but without all of the side effects. Skullcap has an antiinflammatory action and inhibits allergy symptoms by combatting the effects of the histamines. Angelica helps limit the production of allergic antibodies, and licorice is antiinflammatory, as are onions and garlic. These herbal medicines are among those that a naturopath will draw upon in treating allergy.

Working with Your Naturopath   Naturopaths have a holistic approach to the treatment of asthma, as with other ailments. The treatment program will include diet modifi-cation to help you detoxify, avoidance of allergens, and also exercise. Counseling, meditation, and other stress re-duction techniques may also be recommended. Herbal remedies may or may not be part of your treatment.

If you are currently under the care of a medical doctor for your asthma condition, have a talk with him or her about any naturopathic remedies you are considering. It is important always to keep in mind that asthma can in cer-tain circumstances quickly escalate into a life-threatening condition. The medications you are currently taking may be preventing these situations, and suddenly discontinuing them may have results you weren't expecting. Also make sure your naturopath is aware of any other treatment you are receiving from your physician, because many prescrip-tions contain herbs, and these may interfere with any herbal medicines that the naturopath might prescribe.

Nutrition

Asthma is often the result of allergic rhinitis and hay fever, but asthma can also be triggered by a range of other factors, including food allergy. On the positive side, a careful evaluation of your potential food allergies, through medical tests, can help to establish the connection between what you are eating and your asthma. A nutritionist can also help.

Working with a nutritionist, and using the elimination diet, can also help you to discover what foods cause asthma. The elimination diet is described in Chapter 2. While the elimination diet can be a long and time-consuming process, with extensive record keeping as many of the foods you are accustomed to eating are withdrawn and gradually reintroduced, it is an excellent means of discovering what foods you need to avoid while also creating a diet that really works for you. Without going through this process, it is difficult to know what foods may be contributing to your asthma.

There is no magic list of asthma-causing foods. However, some foods are often associated with asthma. For example, eggs are known to produce asthma symptoms. A diet that is heavy in salt, as well as monosodium glutamate (MSG), can also trigger asthma symptoms. Canned soup and soup mixes and packaged food are often prepared with large amounts of salt and MSG. Sulfur dioxide, which is often used as a preservative on the vegetables found in salad bars, in dried fruits, and in seafood, can cause asthma symptoms that, for some people, can be life threatening. Other additives, like food coloring, have been known to be an asthma trigger. While these are a few substances to watch out for, your asthma triggers are unique to you, and may include foods that are not among the usual suspects.

Nutrition is not a miracle cure for asthma, and you should not use your diet as a substitute for medical care. Make sure you communicate with your medical doctor as you make changes to your diet, to make sure that you are not adding or subtracting foods that may adversely affect your overall medical condition. As with allergic conditions, however, eating a balanced diet that is relatively free of preservatives and other chemicals can help keep your body in peak condition.

Reflexology

Reflexology, which is described in Chapter 3, can be helpful both in relieving asthma symptoms as well as rejuvenating the respiratory system and promoting relaxation. The reflex areas that correspond to the lungs are located both in the hands and in the feet. On the hands, the lung reflex areas are on the palms, just below the middle finger and the ring finger. The lung reflex areas on the feet are located on the balls of the feet, below the second, third, and fourth toes, as well as on the tops of the feet, in these same positions.

Working with a reflexologist on a regular basis can help keep your lungs healthy and strong, and even help the lungs to rejuvenate any tissue that may have been damaged as a result of constant infections or pneumonia. Here are some reflexology exercises you can use to strengthen your lungs.

The Hands   Because you have two lungs, the lung reflex area on the right hand corresponds with the right lung, and the same area on the left hand with the left lung. Keep this in mind as you work with your hands because it's important to keep the energy of the lungs balanced by treating them equally. Use the area on the palm just below the base of the middle and ring fingers, as well as the groove in between them. Place the thumb of the other hand on this area and work the whole reflex area with a firm, circular, rolling motion. Use a slight pressure on the first circular motion, and then gradually increase the pressure for each motion. Repeat this circular motion seven times, then repeat the complete series on the other hand.

The Feet You have a lung reflex area on both feet, and as with the hands, the right foot corresponds with the right lung and the left lung with the left foot. Start with the lung reflex area located on the bottom of the foot, at the base of the second, third, and fourth toes, and include the grooves in between. Start under the second toe, and use your thumb to press in a rolling, circular motion, just as you used on your hands. Using the same motion, move from the area under the second toe toward the fourth toe, so that your pressing covers the whole reflex area. With each circular motion, gradually press harder. Repeat this motion seven times on each foot.

As you do these exercises, visualize yourself in a calm and relaxed setting. Imagine that your lungs are growing stronger and healthier, and that you are breathing out all the toxins trapped inside your body. As you press, inhale, and then exhale as you release pressure.

Shiatsu

Shiatsu is useful in treating asthma, preventing an attack by balancing the energy in the meridians and thus strengthening the vitality of the respiratory system. Shiatsu can also be used to reduce asthma symptoms, relieving congestion and difficulty in breathing, though it is not a substitute for medical treatment, especially during an asthma attack. The shiatsu treatment of asthma is focused on the upper back and shoulders, though as always, massage would also be applied to the other parts of the body to create balance.

Here are some examples of the shiatsu approach to asthma, which you can also try on your own.

When treating asthma, the receiver of the shiatsu treatment generally sits in an upright position to aid in breathing. The giver begins by very gently applying pressure with his or her thumbs to the front of the throat, in the cervical region, to calm the tightness in the bronchial tubes. Needless to say, it is important to do this carefully to avoid further breathing constriction. After this, gentle thumb pressure is applied to the back of the neck.

From here, the area between the shoulder blades, on each side of the spine is massaged, also with the thumbs. The giver then moves outward from the spine, on both sides of the back. This area contains rows of points, and each of these is massaged, up and down through each row, moving outward. Massage is then applied to the front of the body, along the deltoid muscles. This treatment might also include deep-breathing exercises, while the giver massages areas around the shoulders, to restore normal breathing.

Asthma can be a life-threatening condition, and you should not make changes to your standard course of treatment from your medical doctor without first talking with him or her about it. Shiatsu can be very beneficial in promoting relaxation and better breathing, and even a measure of symptom relief, but it is not a replacement for the medicines that you may need to keep your symptoms under better control.

Visualization

Stress can only make your asthma symptoms worse. Visualization helps you to relax at a deep level and, in turn, sends messages to your immune system that it's time to turn the alarm system off. You can use visualization on a regular basis, even daily, to help maintain your sense of calm. And you can also visualize to help reduce the feelings of stress and panic that often accompany asthma symptoms. Visualization is described more fully in Chapter 3.

Here's a visualization to use when you feel asthma symptoms coming on:

As soon as you start to wheeze, find a quiet place, and either sit up in a chair or lie on your back. Begin taking slow, rhythmic breaths to relax. As you breathe, remind yourself that you are feeling relaxed, and that everything is fine.

In your mind, form a picture of the allergens that might be causing your asthma symptoms. Think of them floating through the air, and give them a shape, and a color. Watch them coming toward you, and then floating into your nostrils and your mouth as you breathe. As they pass into your system, imagine them causing you to wheeze, sticking in your lungs, and making it harder for you to breathe.

Now turn the tables on your allergens. Imagine that they suddenly turn another color, but it's a peaceful, harmless color. They are still in your system, but they are not there to do damage. In fact, they're telling your body not to worry and fight back, but to relax.

Once you've neutralized the allergens, imagine them gradually floating back out of your body. Feel your bronchial tubes begin to relax, open wider and wider as air passes through. The need to wheeze is passing. Your nasal passages and lungs are relaxing.

Now remind yourself that you are calm and relaxed, and ready to go on with your day.

You may want to practice saying this visualization aloud, and even tape-record your own voice saying it. This way, you'll be able to use it at will to place yourself in a state of calm when you feel symptoms impinging on you. Your reactions to these stressful situations will be both positive and empowered. And with asthma, meeting the symptoms head-on, with relaxation, is one of your best defenses. Use visualization to harness your own natural healing powers.

Yoga

Yoga is the Sanscrit word for "reunion," which refers to the harmony between body and mind. One of the most popular yoga systems, hatha yoga, stresses the importance of body and mind awareness, and teaches various breathing and relaxation techniques to achieve this awareness. Hatha yoga techniques include deep, lung-expanding breathing. Your whole body, including your emotions, may go on "red alert" when asthma symptoms begin to develop, and yoga can help you to become more relaxed as well as breathe better.

Here's an example of one of the more basic hatha yoga breathing exercises:

1. Sit in an upright position, either in a straight-back chair or on a comfortable floor mat.
2. Close your eyes and relax, calming your mind with pleasant thoughts and listening to your breathing.
3. Push all the air out of your lungs by exhaling forcefully.
4. Inhale deeply, but slowly, through your nose. Fill your stomach with air, then your chest, until the air reaches your shoulders.
5. Exhale slowly, pushing the air out first from your shoulders, your chest, and finally from your

stomach. Make sure you have forced out all the air.

6. Repeat this exercise once or twice more.

Yoga teaches you to take calm, deep breaths, providing your lungs with needed exercise. When you feel an allergic reaction coming on, these yoga exercises can help you to remain calm and keep breathing normally.

You can learn hatha techniques by picking up one of the many books on the market and teaching yourself the basics. Books can show you enough to get started on the breathing exercises. However, how you position your body during yoga is a key to gaining the benefits. For example, if you are slumping over too much, or not holding in the oxygen long enough, yoga won't do you a whole lot of good. It may even hurt you if, for example, you have back problems. Or you may pull a muscle.

Yoga classes are available in most communities, through yoga centers, community education programs, and even the YMCA or YWCA. Cost for a series of yoga classes is minimal. Check out the resources in your area and consider signing up for a class, so that a trained instructor is available to guide you in learning the body positions and breathing. With some dedication on your part, you can experience the benefits of yoga—enhanced peace of mind and better breathing—right away.

Meditation and visualization are good practices to supplement yoga.

CHAPTER SEVEN

Juvenile Asthma

Approximately eight million children in the United States have experienced bronchial difficulties on at least one occasion, and two million of these children have chronic asthma. These children are going back and forth to physicians, spending time in the hospital, missing school . . . and keeping their parents up nights listening to their coughing and wheezing, and worrying about them. If you are the parent of an asthmatic child, you probably have a few horror stories of nights spent watching over your own child. And you may have some stories from your own asthmatic childhood.

Chapter 7 provides you with a range of natural treatments for juvenile asthma. The causes and symptoms of juvenile asthma are similar to those of adults—you may want to review Chapter 6, which discusses adult asthma.

WHERE IT ALL BEGINS

Juvenile asthma generally develops before a child's fifth birthday, often between the ages of one and three. Most asthmatic children have experienced an episode of asthma before the age of three, though it may go undiagnosed until a few years later, which makes it difficult to pinpoint exactly when asthma actually occurs in many children.

More boys than girls develop asthma during these early years, though by adolescence the occurrence of asthma in both boys and girls is about the same. The general assumption held by many in the general public is that children outgrow asthma sometime during adolescence. If you're an asthma sufferer, think about your own experience with this ailment. Did you suffer as a child only to have it disappear during high school? Or did your asthma subside for a few years—go undercover—only to return with a vengeance at a later time? The current view of asthma is that children don't actually outgrow it. It may indeed remain dormant for a few years, during a totally unpredictable period of time, and then return during adulthood. Many experts in the field are now saying that the children most likely to outgrow their asthma are boys without additional allergy problems who develop asthma symptoms between the ages of three and eight. Asthma developed before the age of three, or after the age of ten, and with additional allergies, is most likely a lifelong condition, though symptoms during adulthood are often less severe than during childhood.

Triggers of Juvenile Asthma

There are a lot of similarities between childhood and adult asthma; however the same asthma triggers can result in different symptoms in adults and children. For example, a viral infection can cause an allergic reaction in both adults and children. However, the reaction in a child may include more swelling in the airways than in an adult, with more mucus. And because a child's respiratory system is less developed than that of an adult, this swelling can be especially dangerous.

Allergens While the asthma of many adults is not triggered by allergens, at least half of asthmatic children develop asthma symptoms when exposed to allergens, particularly food, pollen, and indoor inhalants like dust. Furthermore, allergens, as well as viral infection, have different effects on children within specific age groups. Infants are most susceptible to viral infection and, to a lesser extent, foods and indoor inhalants. Children from two to six years old are most susceptible to viral infection and indoor inhalants, and less susceptible to foods and pollens. Between the ages of six to twelve, asthma tends to be provoked more by indoor inhalants, pollens, and other irritants, and less by viral infection and food. And during adolescence, asthma tends to be set off by a range of irritants, as well as indoor inhalants and pollen, and to a lesser extent viral infection and food.

Viral Infection Viral infection is a trigger for asthma, particularly in children under the age of three. Most likely, viruses damage the cells that line the airways, which irritates the receptors that lie underneath these cells. The result is the wheezing commonly associated with an episode of asthma. Some experts have found that a viral infection can also lead to the first development of allergy symptoms.

Foods Food allergies are common in both adults and children. However, a food allergy is much more likely to cause asthma symptoms in a child than in an adult. The main reason for this difference is that the digestive tracts of children are still under development, and they do not digest food as easily. While a range of foods can trigger juvenile asthma symptoms, cow's milk and eggs are the ones most likely. Breast-feeding during the first six months of life can help prevent allergy, and is a good precaution if you have a history of milk allergies in your family.

Inhalants Inhaled allergens, such as dust, mold, pollen, and animal dander can cause asthma during the early childhood years, i.e., after the age of two. During infancy, inhalants are less of a concern.

Exercise Asthmatic children commonly overreact to exercise. Of particular concern is exercise that places continual strain on the respiratory system, such as running or riding a bicycle for long distances. Team sports, like baseball, are less likely to present problems because participants are provided with periods of rest during the course of a game.

Environmental Irritants Environmental irritants like cigarette smoke, chemicals, car exhaust, and other air pollution irritate the airways of asthmatic children.

Psychological Factors in Juvenile Asthma

Feelings and thoughts that are held inside will come out one way or another, often expressed as physical symptoms, and it's important for parents of asthmatic children to pay close attention to how their children feel about themselves.

Asthmatic children cannot always participate in sports and other physical activities, and they often feel as though they are not "like the other kids," resulting in feelings of low self-esteem and alienation. When other children refer to them as weak, and different, children begin to embrace these labels. When we don't feel good about ourselves, at any age, our physical vitality and health can suffer.

Feelings of stress, either at home or at school, often

lead to feelings of fear and panic. For asthmatic children there is a direct relationship between these feelings and asthma symptoms. And difficulty in breathing can lead to even more fear and panic until it becomes an endless cycle.

Asthmatic children have what seems like a built-in system for emotional expression. Some experts point to a close link between emotions and asthma, and it has been theorized that asthmatic children express their anger by having asthma attacks that not only scare the adults around them but also gain them attention. However, many other experts disagree with this theory, calling it not only an unfair criticism of children who are already suffering from a debilitating condition but also an oversimplification of the complex nature of asthma. And most important, a child who is having an asthma attack does need immediate, and sometimes emergency, attention, regardless of what the causes appear to be.

Caution: Asthma Can Be Life Threatening

Asthma can be a life-threatening condition, and symptoms can occur and progress at frightening speed. If your child has asthma, he or she should be under the care of a medical doctor who has prescribed any necessary medication and briefed you on how to handle an emergency.

Use natural medicine alternatives as a means of keeping asthma symptoms at bay, as well as a means of coping with asthma symptoms when they do occur. However, do not experiment with your child's health. Talk with your medical doctor about alternatives, and make sure any alternatives you use will not interfere with your child's regular medical care.

NATURAL TREATMENTS FOR JUVENILE ASTHMA

Acupressure

Because of its focus on effective breathing, acupressure treatment can be especially helpful in treating children with asthma. With parental supervision, older children can learn exercises that involve using the acupressure points to strengthen the lungs and relieve asthma symptoms as they occur. While some of the exercises may be too complicated for children to undertake on their own, others are so simple that children can begin to relieve their own symptoms when their parents aren't around.

To investigate acupressure treatment for children, start with a practitioner who has experience in treating asthmatic children. You'll need to be involved at every step, observing and even assisting with each session so that you and your child work as a team in learning each exercise. Make sure your child understands the purpose of acupressure exercises and talks about how he or she feels during the exercises as well as afterward. If pain or any other negative effects are reported, the practitioner will need to make adjustments.

Affirmations

An asthma attack can be a terrifying experience for a child, and the panic that often results can make the symptoms seem even more severe. Children panic during an allergy attack, and they are often not sophisticated enough to use techniques like meditation to calm themselves. This is where affirmations can help.

Experience teaches children that once an asthma attack begins, it will be a scary experience with wheezing and difficulty in breathing. Affirmations can calm the panic that accompanies these symptoms, replacing negative self-talk with messages of strength, good health, and calmness. Affirmations can be a form of self-hypnosis in this sense, said over and over like a mantra to focus attention away from the illness.

Here are a few affirmations to use with asthmatic children.

- I don't have to be afraid.
- I am strong and healthy.
- My lungs are clear and I can breathe.
- I am getting better every day.
- My wheezing will go away soon.

Parents and children can work together to create affirmations and turn it into a game by writing them down on sheets of paper that can be hung on the bedroom wall, and even drawing pictures to illustrate them. Try practicing affirmations before school, maybe during breakfast, and again before bedtime. And always use them during an asthma attack to help induce a sense of calm control.

Aromatherapy

Aromatherapy, described in depth in Chapter 4, can also be used in relieving the symptoms of juvenile asthma. An aroma lamp, for example, can be placed in a child's room, permeating the room with aromas that promote health and help to quell the symptoms of allergy. While you will want to avoid placing an open flame in a child's room, lamps that use light bulbs can both be fun and serve as a night-light. Children love smelling the fresh fragrances. Compresses soaked in water and essential oils can relieve chest congestion. The use of aromatherapy with children is discussed in Chapter 5, Juvenile Allergies.

Aromatherapy helps to reduce the effects of asthma in much the same way as with adults. The aromas from the essential oils counteract the effects of allergenic inhalants by stimulating the relief-giving and health-enhancing neurotransmitters of the central nervous system. Children's systems are more sensitive than adults, and they will not require as many drops of whatever oil you are using.

The essential oils that children seem to respond to best include tangerine, orange, cinnamon, and vanilla. Placing one of these scents in a child's room will promote calm, a sense of well-being, and general good health. You may want to read your child a special story as these scents permeate the room.

The following are suggested applications of aromatherapy for relieving juvenile asthma:

Congestion Essential oils used in an aroma lamp can relieve congestion by acting as an expectorant and decongestant. The essential oils to use include eucalyptus, pine, lemon, myrtle, and naiouli. Just two drops of these oils, which is about half the adult dose, is enough.

Cough Hyssop is also a good remedy for the wheezing and coughing associated with asthma, because it helps to heal the bronchial passages. Add a couple of drops to an aroma lamp, especially at night. Hyssop also works well with lemon oil, which has a regenerative effect. Hyssop can be taken internally but this is not recommended for children. However, a few drops can be rubbed on the chest, as a salve.

Wheezing and Difficult Breathing The essential oil of eucalyptus aids the breathing process by helping to regenerate lung tissue while also acting as an expectorant, decongestant, and cough suppressant. Use a child-sized amount, two drops, in an electric aroma lamp, both during the day and at night.

Children often experience fear and panic during an asthma attack, and this can increase the tightness in the chest. Essential oils like lavender have a regenerative effect on the nervous system and thus promote a feeling of calm. Place a drop or two in the aroma lamp. A couple of drops may also be taken orally for the same effect.

Aromatherapy works well with other natural treatments. For example, if you are teaching your child to visualize or use affirmations, practicing these techniques in a room with an aroma lamp and a few drops of essential oils can enhance the process. Check with your physician or other practitioner, however, before you give your child a cough syrup based on essential oils, particularly if another one has been prescribed. Additionally, if your child has any negative reactions to the essential oils, discontinue their use. Keep in mind that essential oils can have toxic side effects, and these effects can be much more pronounced in children. Always keep essential oils out of the reach of young children.

Botanical Medicine

Herbal preparations have historically been used in treating the wheezing, coughing, and chest congestion associated with asthma. And because many of these preparations are used externally, rather than ingested, they can be considered safe for use with children. Botanical medicine is described in more depth in Chapter 4. The botanical medicine approach to childhood allergies is similar to that of adult allergies in that the starting place for treatment is through detoxification of the system to rid it of impurities, followed by the treatment of specific symptoms, and then strengthening the weakened areas.

Compresses and salves made with herbs can be placed on a child's chest for a short period of time or even overnight to help relieve asthma symptoms. Herbs can also be ingested in weak teas. When working with children, use herbs carefully. Greatly dilute the standard adult dose, even when the herbs are being used externally, because a child's skin is much more sensitive than that of an adult and thus more prone to irritation. Don't use herbs internally without working with a practitioner who has experience in treating children. Also keep in mind that the use of herbs can affect the medical treatment your child may be receiving, especially since many medications are derived from herbs. Consult with your pediatrician to make sure he or she is aware of this treatment and supports it.

Children can benefit from the use of herbs in treating their asthma. Herbs stimulate a child's own natural defenses and further strengthen the system without adding the synthetic chemicals, alcohol, sugar, food dye, and other additives that are often found in cough medicines. Herbs also have strengthening and restorative effects on children. They can be used to make the respiratory system healthier, strengthening the lungs so that your child is less susceptible to and debilitated by the effects of asthma. For example, the tendency toward congestion and mucus production can be reduced. Furthermore, herbs can have a relaxing effect, which in turn reduces hypersensitivity and the panic reaction that often accompanies an asthma attack. Here are a few herbal treatments for juvenile allergy that you can try at home.

Congestion   Congestion and mucus production can be relieved by a compress using ginger. Mix a few drops of a tincture of ginger, which you can purchase from a health food store, with four tablespoons of whole wheat flour and enough water to make a paste. Spread it on a piece of cotton cloth, and then lay it over your child's chest. Leave it on for at least an hour.

Congestion and cough can also be relieved by using a tea made of gingerroot. Follow these directions for making ginger tea:

1. Grate two inches of gingerroot.
2. Place it in a teapot.
3. Boil one quart of water, and then pour it over the ginger.
4. Cover the teapot and let it steep at least fifteen minutes.
5. Drink it warm or cool.

Serve the ginger tea to your child a few times per day, or until the symptoms disappear.

To relieve your child's congestion and dry out excess mucus, try a mixture of the powders of ginger, black pepper, and aniseed. Combine small amounts of each of these powders—perhaps a pinch of each for a child's dose—and combine it with either warm milk or a teaspoon of honey. This mixture is taken internally. Check with your practitioner before administering this remedy to a child.

Cough   The coughing associated with asthma can be treated by a mixture of herbal oils, which you can purchase at a health food store. Combine an ounce each of the herbal oils of cinnamon, eucalyptus, thyme, camphor, and marjoram. Also add a few drops of olive oil to dilute this mixture and store it in a bottle. Spread it on your child's chest at bedtime—it will have a healing and soothing action that will help relieve a hacking cough and associated congestion.

You can also rub a small amount of eucalyptus oil into your child's chest, before bed, to help relieve coughing.

Using Herbal Treatments for Juvenile Asthma
When treating your child with herbs, there are a few rules of thumb to keep in mind. First and foremost, as mentioned previously, work with a practitioner, with the approval of your pediatrician. Use greatly reduced amounts of each herb. If your practitioner has recommended using an herb internally, and your child complains about the taste of the herb, do not force it on him or her. Try chopping it up in a spoonful of honey or peanut butter. Watch closely for reactions, as well as improvement. If your child's symptoms worsen, or if your child seems to be having a reaction of any severity, discontinue use and seek medical attention. Also watch to make sure any salves or compresses you use are not reddening, burning, or otherwise irritating your child's skin. And if you don't see any improvement in your child's condition within a few days, check with your practitioner. Unless the herb was intended to gradually strengthen and nurture your child's natural defenses, it may not be working.

Botanical medicine should not be used with aromatherapy or homeopathy.

Breathing Exercises

The importance of strong, healthy lungs cannot be emphasized enough. For asthmatic children, simply reminding them that they need to breathe deeply is not enough; they need help in learning to take deep breaths, and remembering to keep their lungs exercised through constant practice. Parents can help here.

Chapter 6, which focuses on adult asthma, includes a set of breathing exercises. These exercises can also be used with children, under adult supervision. Talk with your medical doctor about how best to proceed with these exercises and then, with your doctor's permission, begin practicing them with your child, preferably on a daily basis. This can become part of an afterschool or evening routine, and even a game.

Exercise

Asthmatic children often feel like wallflowers because they are unable to participate in normal games and activities that other children are enjoying. While these activities may indeed be too strenuous, asthmatic children can often participate on a modified basis. And with the availability of adequate medication and watchful supervision by an adult who has been educated about asthma, asthmatic children can often participate along with the other children. This is certainly better than sitting on the sidelines out of fear of having an asthma attack.

Talk with your child's medical doctor about what precautions to take before and during physical activity. For example, strenuous play in very cold weather or on a dusty gym floor may either require additional medication or other precautions. Work with your child's physical education teacher or an exercise consultant to find activities at which your asthmatic child can excel. Most of all, talk with your child about preferred activities and how much he or she would like to participate

With careful planning, and much encouragement, your child can be participating in many of the same activities as other children. This will enhance your child's physical health, strengthen lung capacity, and work wonders for self-esteem.

Homeopathy

Homeopathy can be helpful when applied to juvenile asthma. However, just as homeopathic physicians are particularly cautious when treating children, they approach the treatment of asthma with extreme caution. Juvenile asthma, when accompanied by congested and labored breathing, can be a dangerous condition. While a young child's immune system and natural defenses are under development, and conventional medicines can both short-circuit development and cover symptoms, this medicine may also prevent death. For this reason practitioners recognize the need for conventional medications and the ongoing care of a physician to assure that emergency care is readily available in the event of a serious asthma attack.

While being extremely cautious, homeopathic physicians do offer assistance to children with asthma. These remedies can help to strengthen the respiratory system, as well as provide relief for mild wheezing and congestion. Homeopathic care begins at home. When asthma-related wheezing is minor, and the breathing is not seriously labored, practitioners first recommend that you give your child plenty of liquids. Rapid breathing depletes the body of water, and drinking a lot of water helps to replace liquids, while also helping to loosen the mucus that is clogging up breathing passages. Simple breathing exercises, discussed earlier, will also help strengthen the lungs and aid in relaxation.

Treating Your Child's Asthma with Homeopathy Homeopathy may not be able to cure your child's asthma. This condition, as discussed earlier in this chapter, may be the result of a range of factors, including genetic inheritance. However, even with chronic asthma, your child most likely experiences periods of time in which he or she is relatively free of asthma symptoms. Homeopathy can help your child to extend these periods of better health by building up his or her constitution, and offering relief from minor symptoms.

Chamomilla   Chamomilla, derived from chamomile, is an especially child-friendly homeopathic medicine, and is useful in a range of childhood illnesses such as colic as well as asthma. Children who may benefit from chamomilla are irritable and given to anger, demanding, and stubbornly disagreeable. These emotions can also contribute to asthma symptoms. Thus, chamomilla is administered to children primarily as a result of these behaviors, though asthma symptoms may also be present. Once the chamomilla has helped to bring these symptoms under control, the wheezing and other asthma symptoms may also subside, or even be prevented.

When administering chamomilla to a child, give him or her a single dose, and watch for an improvement in behavior. Follow this with hourly doses, and then space them out over a few hours. Watch for changes and be ready to seek emergency care if indicated. Do not exceed ten doses over two days.

Arsenicum Album   If chamomilla is not helpful in relieving your child's asthma symptoms, you may also want to try arsenicum, which is the most commonly used homeopathic medicine for asthma. Symptoms that are a match for arsenicum include feelings of fearfulness and restfulness, often related to the panic that many asthmatics experience when they cannot breathe adequately. The asthma symptoms most likely worsen at night, with wheezing and congestion increasing to the point that your child tosses and turns, and constantly gets up to take deep breaths. Weakness may also accompany these symptoms, as well as a cough, chills, and thirst. Even if these symptoms do not noticeably worsen at night, arsenicum may still be helpful.

Pulsatilla Pulsatilla, derived from windflower, is an alternate medicine for asthma. This choice is in part based on behaviors that include being unusually affectionate or tearful and afraid of being left alone. Asthma-related symptoms indicating a compatibility with pulsatilla include wheezing that either begins or worsens during the evening and night. Coughing accompanied by the need to bring up phlegm that has accumulated in the chest is another symptom, as is a worsening of symptoms after eating.

Ipecac If your child's asthma symptoms include a large amount of phlegm in the chest, ipecac is the recommended homeopathic medicine. Symptoms associated with a need for ipecac may include extreme wheezing, accompanied by a rattling of mucus deep within the chest. The presence of mucus is also obvious during coughing, which can become so intense that your child starts gagging and vomiting. Nausea may also be present as well as exhaustion, and a pale and sickly appearance. Be careful here: A phlegmy cough can also be a symptom of pneumonia, a condition to which asthmatic children are particularly susceptible. Always report this situation to a medical doctor.

Spongia Asthma symptoms that do not include phlegm, but instead a dryness, often evidenced by a harsh, unproductive cough, indicate a need for Spongia, which is derived from roasted sponge. Other symptoms associated with a need for Spongia are noisy and labored breathing with a whistling sound. These symptoms may come after being chilled or having a cold. Wheezing may worsen during sleep, with breathing becoming more labored when lying down. Wheezing may lessen after a warm drink.

It almost goes without saying that if you administer homeopathic medicine to treat your child's asthma, do it carefully and only after consulting with your pediatrician. Start with single doses, with the first three doses given every two hours, then discontinued as soon as there is some improvement. If there is no improvement after the third dose, wait an hour and try a new medicine, also following it with two additional doses every two hours. Don't use these medicines more than once in two hours, and don't use more than ten doses in two days.

As a rule of thumb, treat juvenile asthma only under the guidance of a homeopathic practitioner.

Working with a Homeopathic Physician Your child's asthma symptoms can change and worsen quickly. These symptoms can cause severe respiratory distress and even fatality, especially in young children. Use homeopathic medicine under the guidance of a practitioner, and stay in close contact, even on a daily basis, when you are in the midst of using a medicine to treat specific symptoms. Let him or her know how the medicines are affecting your child, so that changes can be made quickly. As always, if your child experiences a sudden change in symptoms, including severe shortness of breath or a sore throat with difficulty in swallowing, contact a medical doctor immediately.

Making your own diagnosis of your child's asthma is both difficult and unwise. Your child may not be able to report exactly how he or she is feeling, and in most cases,

you have to rely on your own observations. While you can
discontinue a medicine if it does not seem to be helping,
you may waste time with remedies that are not working.
And while wasting time, you may also be allowing your
child's symptoms to worsen dangerously.

A homeopathic physician can help you to avoid these
mistakes. He or she will begin by carefully examining your
child, while asking you and your child a detailed list of
questions about how and when the symptoms occur and
the conditions surrounding these situations. You will be
called on to provide detailed information about your
child's likes and dislikes, emotional makeup, mental and
intellectual state, and history of childhood illnesses. You
may want to bring the baby book along. Also, keep a journal of how your child has behaved in the days before and
after an allergy attack, including food, hours of sleep, and
the specific symptoms. This information will all be used by
the homeopathic practitioner in choosing an initial course
of treatment.

Try to work with a homeopathic physician who is also a
medical doctor, preferably one who has experience in
working with asthmatic children. He or she will be most
qualified to assess the symptoms and set up a treatment
program that not only helps to relieve your child's symptoms, but also helps build up his or her system to withstand future attacks. Remember that homeopathic medicine may not be able to provide a total cure.

If your homeopathic physician is not also a medical
doctor, you should let your physician know that your child
is being treated with homeopathic remedies. He or she
can still provide you with medicines to use in the event of
severe asthma symptoms, and can also serve as the first
contact in the case of an emergency. And in the event of
any kind of medical emergency, contact your physician to
provide emergency treatment and arrange for hospitaliza-

tion if needed. Many physicians accept the validity of natural approaches and will work with you and your practitioner. Homeopathy can also be supplemented by exercises to help your child breathe better.

Naturopathy

Naturopaths treat juvenile asthma in much the same way as adult asthma, with some differences, and many cautions. Naturopaths look to three major causes in determining the factors that lead to asthma. Naturopaths view juvenile asthma as related to, and even an outcome of, childhood allergies, including food allergy, allergic rhinitis, and eczema. A low stomach acidity is another factor recognized by naturopaths in the development of allergic rhinitis and hay fever, with food staying in the stomach longer and creating imbalances that lead to allergic reactions and then asthma. Additionally, children with asthma have a defect in a chemical called leukotrienes that aids in the creation of serotonin, which in turn is a broncho-constricting agent; this can be treated with a vitamin B_6 supplement.

Exposure to food additives is also viewed by naturopaths as one of the causes of asthma. Artificial dyes and preservatives like sulfur dioxide are used in packaged foods and drinks.

Treating Asthma with Naturopathy   Naturopaths advocate avoiding the use of drugs in treating children. Antibiotics are viewed as throwing off the digestive tract, for example, and drugs like cortisone displace symptoms from one area of the body to another. Thus, naturopaths treat asthma primarily through diet, and for asthmatics they recommended a vegetarian diet. This includes avoiding all meat, fish, dairy products, and eggs, and drinking spring water. Soda and other stimulants, as well as sugar and salt, must be avoided. This diet does include unlimited amounts of vegetables, including lettuce, broccoli, celery, beets, cucumber and most beans except soy and green beans. Restricted amounts of potatoes are allowed, with most fruits except apples and citrus fruits, and very restricted amounts of grains.

Animal fats help to produce leukotrienes, which in turn stimulate the bronchial constriction response, and a vegetarian diet eliminates these leukotrienes from the diet. This diet should lead to improvement of symptoms after approximately four months, though it may be necessary to stay on it for a year or more. The benefit of this diet is that it eliminates the allergens that are being consumed through the food, resulting in a gradual detoxification.

Nutritional supplements are often used in treating asthma. Vitamin B_6 can help decrease the number of asthma attacks, and cause them to be less severe. Vitamin B_{12} helps prevent asthma symptoms brought on by exposure to sulfites. Vitamin C helps to prevent severe bronchial constriction, and may even help to prevent attacks, as well as serve as a possible defense against allergens. Carotenes strengthen the lining of the respiratory track, while vitamin E is antiinflammatory. Naturopaths vary in their use of supplements and vitamins in treating asthma; however it is not uncommon for a practitioner to prescribe one or more from this group as a component of treatment.

Naturopaths will also recommend the use of botanical medicines in treating asthma. These medicines include Ephedra, which acts as an antiinflammatory and antiallergy agent. The usefulness of Ephedra diminishes if it is used repeatedly over time, and it is often supplemented by other herbs, like licorice, as well as vitamin C, vitamin B_6, and other nutritional supplements. Ephedra is often used with herbal expectorants like licorice or senega to help clear the respiratory tract of mucus. The herbal medicine skullcap is similar in effect to drugs like aspirin and ibuprofen, but without all of the side effects. Skullcap has an antiinflammatory action, and inhibits allergy symptoms by combatting the effects of the histamines.

Working with Your Naturopath The naturopathic approach to promoting good health can be helpful in treating an asthmatic child. Watching your child's eating habits—avoiding sugar, bleached flour, and preservatives, and choosing food from the major food groups—can have pronounced benefits for your child's health. Vitamin supplements can enhance vitality.

If your child suffers from asthma, you are most likely working with a medical doctor who is prescribing medications as well as serving as an emergency contact. Let your physician know whatever you are doing with naturopathic treatment, so that he or she can in turn advise you about the implications of mixing whatever medicines your child may be taking with the vitamins or herbal remedies that your naturopath may prescribe.

Also keep in mind that sudden changes in diet can be stressful to a child who already feels like an outsider due to his or her illness. Introduce diet changes slowly, and present your child with as many food choices as possible so that he or she feels some measure of control over this aspect of life. Make it as much fun as you can, with interesting recipe variations and by letting your child help you in the kitchen.

Nutrition

Good nutrition is important for asthmatic children. A diet that is heavy in food additives, like preservatives, adds more toxins to their systems, interfering with the development of their natural defenses against illness. Also, additives like sulfites can bring on asthma attacks and can be life threatening.

Furthermore, weight control is important with asthmatic children. Excess weight makes it harder for them to participate in daily activities, adds to their self-image as outsiders, and strains the heart and lungs.

The best diet for asthmatic children is one that includes adequate portions from all of the food groups, as described in Chapter 3. Additionally, all food additives should be avoided as much as possible, especially those to which the child is known to be allergic. Also, carefully monitor the consumption of dairy products, since these add to the production of mucus, which leads to increased congestion.

Psychotherapy

Children suffering from asthma experience a wide range of emotions in relation to their illness. Sometimes it is clear what they are feeling—rage, for example, or sadness. Other times, children can be hard to read, either because they won't say what's on their mind or they don't have the vocabulary to draw on. One certainty, however, is that they have a range of thoughts, feelings, and perceptions about their illness. And while it is both unfair and dangerous to simply say that a child has asthma because of emotional problems or, worse yet, because the child wants to be sick, the emotional aspect of asthma can't be ignored.

If you have an asthmatic child, you may have wondered how he or she is feeling inside. Does your child feel accepted and equal to his or her brothers and sisters, or unique, or more like a burden? When he or she gets upset, is it possible for the child to be expressive, or do the asthma symptoms come on too fast? Or does your child seem so unemotional that you don't see any response at all? And also remember that outside of your house, your child lives in another world of competitive and sometimes cruel children and insensitive teachers. He or she may feel like an outsider in that world.

While you may feel you have done your best to provide an open relationship with your child, he or she may feel uncomfortable talking about emotions directed at you. Or if there are problems at school, your child may feel as if he or she would be letting you down by telling you about them.

Child psychotherapy helps to resolve emotional conflicts that might be a factor in asthma, with the therapist acting as a neutral third party, meeting with your child on a regular basis to talk about home and school. Each therapist works differently, and will view your child as presenting a unique set of concerns, so it is difficult to know ahead of time exactly what will occur in a therapy session.

Generally, a child psychotherapist will use talk therapy with your child, meeting once or more per week for about an hour. During this time, the talking will center around how your child is feeling about the people in his or her life, at school and at home. The session may involve playing games or drawing pictures, even watching videotapes, all of which are used by the therapist to understand your child and how best to offer help. Most likely, the therapist will discuss new ways of coping with emotions and techniques for responding differently to situations as they arise.

The process of therapy can last weeks, months, and even years. And to a great extent, you will know it is working with your child only by what you observe in his or her behavior, as well as what you feel in your own "gut." After a relatively short period of time, even a few weeks, you may be able to observe some positive change. However, keep in mind that sometimes children act out new emotions and exhibit new behaviors that may not be what you had hoped to see. Give the therapy time to work, and allow your child to make behavior changes at his or her own pace.

When you are choosing a child psychotherapist, make sure you find one who has extensive experience in working with asthmatic children. You can obtain names of therapists through your local mental health clinic, community hospital, or university. You may also want to ask acquaintances for a recommendation. Choose a therapist with whom you feel comfortable as a parent so that you can voice concerns as they arise, though the therapist may not want to discuss the specific content of each session.

Reflexology

You can use reflexology with a child to promote relaxation, as well as to relieve asthma symptoms. But the benefits of using reflexology techniques with your asthmatic child are also psychological, and even spiritual, and they can have a profound effect on helping your child manage his or her asthma symptoms. Reflexology is described in Chapter 3.

Reflexology opens up a whole new means of communication between you and your child, a communication without words, with you as the giver and your child as the receiver. This can be especially helpful during those times when your child is feeling upset, angry, or fearful, and either doesn't know how to express these feelings or is afraid of how you will react. Also, asthmatic children often feel different and alienated from the people around them. With reflexology your child can relax while you show your feelings and concern—you focus your love on each other in ways that can't be expressed in words.

As your child grows older, you may want to teach him or her a few reflexology techniques, so that you can also be on the receiving end from time to time.

A reflexology practitioner can help you to develop a set of reflexology exercises that work especially well with children, and suggest ways to develop a routine that will work well with your child's symptoms. Here's an example of how you can use reflexology with your child at home.

Thumb Walking   Thumb walking is helpful in breaking up congestion and relaxing the muscles around the bronchial tubes. Use the outer edge of your thumb, near the tip, while bending your thumb only at the top joint. Do the thumb walking on the fleshy areas on the soles of your child's feet, with a steady and even pressure. Use your other fingers on top of the foot to hold it in place. Start at the base of the heel, making small presses as if you were walking, and gradually move upward to the toes in a straight line. When you reach the toes, start back at the bottom of the foot, moving your thumb over a bit. Cover the whole foot using this method.

Finger Walking   Finger walking helps to break up congestion in the chest. Use the same basic action as in thumb walking, up and down the foot, with the corner edge of the index finger. Bend this finger from the first joint only, while keeping the rest of the index finger straight. Make small presses, beginning at the bottom of the heel, and move upward as if you were walking with your index finger. When you reach the toes, start back at the bottom of the heel and work upward again, as if you were creating rows of lines on the bottom of the foot.

Using Reflexology with Your Asthmatic Child   If your child responds well to reflexology, you may want to make it part of your nightly bedtime routine. Make sure you talk to your child calmly as you try the exercises, to make sure that you are not causing any discomfort. As you become more proficient, a fifteen-minute reflexology session accompanied by a pleasant visualization or a bedtime story can send your child off to sleep feeling relaxed and loved.

While a reflexologist can provide you with other specific asthma-related techniques to use, you can also pick up much of this information in a book. As with other methods of massage, the most important ingredient in applying reflexology is a loving attitude toward the other person, and enough verbal communication to learn what feels good and what does not.

Visualization

Children have active imaginations, and one of the ways they exercise their imaginations is through visualization. You can help your child to harness this ability for use in dealing with the symptoms of asthma. Visualization can be helpful both in preventing asthma as well as in helping to reduce the symptoms of an attack.

Use visualization as if it were a game that you and your child play, especially at night before bedtime. Let your child use his or her imagination to come up with enjoyable, relaxing images, like going for a walk, or riding in a boat, or playing with friends. Teach your child to close his or her eyes and imagine this setting. Ask questions about what it looks like, feels like, and smells like as your child describes this relaxing setting to you. Help your child to understand the connection between a pleasant visualization and the feelings of pleasure and relaxation that accompany it. The next time your child is threatened by asthma symptoms, sit down and guide him or her through this visualization.

Visualization is described in more depth in Chapter 3. You may also want to use the visualizations described in Chapter 6.

CHAPTER EIGHT

Inorganic Allergies and Chronic Industrial Irritants

Whether you are sitting in your house or your car, the air you are taking in may be full of pollution, and this can make you feel miserable. You can also come into contact with chemicals through touching and breathing the fumes from the many household products you use on an average day.

If you find yourself experiencing occasional skin irritations, or nausea and diarrhea, or unexpected coughing or sneezing, these symptoms may be the result of your environment. And the offending toxins may be obvious. For example, an especially hazy, humid, and smoggy day can leave you feeling congested and short of breath. Or a meal of canned or otherwise prepared food, or food from a fast-food restaurant, can bombard your system with a high level of additives. Or a household cleaner can give you an unexpected rash.

We are all living in the center of a toxic environment. If you are allergy prone, these toxins may be making your symptoms even worse. But even if you have always thought of yourself as allergy free, your environment may be presenting you with new challenges, and symptoms. And as always, treatment begins with understanding your symptoms and what's causing them.

A DEFINITION OF INORGANIC
ALLERGIES

Inorganic allergies are those that result from manufactured substances. They are induced by artificial substances, found in, for example, industrial waste and household products. While these substances are everywhere, each individual's levels of tolerance to exposure depend on a wide range of factors, described in a later section. But first, let's take a quick look at the symptoms of inorganic allergies.

Upper Respiratory Symptoms   Upper respiratory symptoms from exposure to industrial irritants can include inflammation of the nasal membranes, sinus problems, coughing, frequent throat clearing, and postnasal drip. The eyes can become itchy.

Lower Respiratory Symptoms   Industrial irritants can cause hoarseness, bronchitis, coughing, and wheezing. If you have a tendency toward asthma, sensitivity to industrial irritants may provoke it.

Skin Reactions   Eczema, hives, and itching can be the result of physical contact with an artificial chemical, such as a dye.

Gastrointestinal Problems   Gastrointestinal symptoms are most likely caused by an allergy to a specific food. These symptoms, however, can also show up after exposure to chemicals such as preservatives. Symptoms include diarrhea, constipation, nausea, bloating, vomiting, and gas.

∘   ∘   ∘

Other symptoms that can result from exposure to an industrial irritant include headaches, muscle aches, fatigue, and depression.

If you are experiencing any of these symptoms, it is important to keep track of when they occur and what kind of an environment you are in at the time. You cannot always avoid the substances that are affecting you. We all have to breathe. However, by being aware of the specific conditions that lead to your allergic reactions, you can better select a treatment.

Who Is Allergic?

Each person has his or her own unique responses to allergens in the environment, with symptoms varying widely. You may find yourself sneezing on an overcast, smoggy day, while a coworker or family member has a severe headache. And you may have no reaction at all on a similar day a week later. These differences in reactions are the result of your unique combination of the following characteristics:

- how allergic you are
- the degree and duration of the exposure
- your age
- your sex
- your heredity
- whether you smoke
- your diet
- your general physical condition
- your environment at home
- your psychological state of mind

If you find yourself reacting more on one day then another, think of what's going on in your life that day. Did you sleep well? Have you been outside a lot? Did you have lunch? Are you feeling calm and relaxed or stressed out? All of these factors combine with circumstances that we have no control over, such as age and heredity, to determine our reactions to the environment.

What Causes Inorganic Allergies

The major causes of inorganic allergies include common household products and air pollution. Each individual reacts to these substances differently or not at all. Below are some examples of these substances.

Household Products   While the chemical industry has provided us with a range of advantages, these benefits have not been without cost. Artificial chemicals in items from clothing to household products have introduced a whole new family of allergies, with many people experiencing allergic reactions who were previously allergy free.

These chemicals are everywhere, waiting to be breathed, touched, or eaten by unsuspecting humans. Spray residues from Alar, for example, contaminate fruits such as peaches, apples, and cherries. During an average growing season, fruit may be sprayed ten or fifteen times, resulting in an extensive saturation of pesticides. Simple washing does not completely rid fruit of these chemical residues. In some individuals, it takes a very small amount of Alar to cause a reaction, with symptoms that include hives, headaches, and asthma. Chemicals such as Alar are also present in vegetables and, due to the spraying of animal feed, they are also present in meat.

Dried fruits and nuts are often fumigated with a chemical called methyl bromide, which also leaves a residue that can result in an allergic reaction with symptoms such as an upset stomach. The use of sulfites as a food preservative is further discussed in Chapter 10.

Examples of artificial chemicals that can cause allergic responses include petrochemicals, halogens, sulfur, and ammonia. Some of the products that contain these chemicals are listed below.

Petrochemicals

perfume
food dyes and additives
synthetic fibers
paint
plastic
adhesives
alcohol
inks
cleaning solvents

Formaldehyde, which is derived from petrochemicals, is a common chemical found in the home. Formaldehyde is used in products that include:

antiperspirants
disinfectants
antiseptics
some nail polishes
preservatives

Formaldehyde is also used in clothing to help make it flameproof, and to keep it from wrinkling and shrinking.

Halogens

chlorine
paper
insecticides
anesthetics
herbicides
drugs
processed foods

Sulfur

dandruff shampoo
food preservatives
photography supplies
wine

Ammonia

disinfectants and cleansers
fertilizers
rubber
fabric dyes
rayon
glue
soap
home-insulating material

If you have developed an allergy to one of these chemicals you may experience allergy symptoms whenever you come into contact with any of the substances that contain it. For example, if you have a petrochemical allergy, you may have a reaction to perfume, synthetic fibers, and certain food additives. As a result, you'll need to be on guard against any of these products.

While skin contact and consumption can lead to a reaction, many chemicals emit a gas that, when breathed by an allergic person, can cause a reaction. Some products are more likely to emit a gas than others. A list of such products compiled by NASA includes the following materials, many of which are found in the average home:

Polyester, found in fabric used in clothing, furniture upholstery, drapery, and in pillow stuffing.

Polyethylenes, used in containers for food.

Polyvinyls, found in leatherlike material used in upholstery, artificial flowers, shower curtains, and electrical conduits.

Silicones, used as a sealant in household appliances, such as refrigerators and dishwashers.

Epoxies, used as a household adhesive and in electronic equipment.

Polyurethanes, used in stuffing pillows and mattresses and in insulation.

Fluorocarbons, used in the Freon gas found in the cooling systems of air-conditioners and refrigerators. These fluorocarbons can often leak into the environment.

A wide range of other common substances can cause allergic reactions. These include:

chlorine
ink
cigarette smoke
natural gas

Air Pollution   The dangers of air pollution have been discussed in the news media for years, and it is generally agreed that breathing the air can be a dangerous proposition. For those with an allergy of one kind or another, air pollution can be even more of a problem. And it is not only outdoor air that can be dangerous, but also the air that circulates indoors.

Petrochemicals are the major culprit, particularly if you are susceptible to petrochemical fumes. First, there is the obvious, like the exhaust from automobiles and buses. The fumes from hydrocarbon fuels such as coal, gasoline, and natural gas can lead to occasional or even chronic illness due to prolonged exposure. And because these fuels are used for indoor heating, the exposure can be nonstop. Old oil tanks may leak, and allow fumes to spread throughout the ventilation system. Oil tanks can also overflow while they are being filled, and fuel that ends up on the floor of a basement can give off fumes for weeks and months.

Natural gas, though it is considered to be less smog producing than other fuels, can also lead to allergic reactions. Natural gas is delivered at higher pressures than other fuels, so a microscopic leak in a fuel line can allow fumes to escape into the air. Furthermore, a gas stove can be a source of irritation, even if the gas has been turned off, as some uncombusted gas leaks from any gas stove in the seconds between turning the valve and having the pilot light catch and, over several years, this can leave a residue lingering in your environment.

Furnaces not only circulate fumes from fuel but dust collects in furnaces and this dust is also spread throughout a house or office building.

The pesticides used on plants are circulated in the air. Pesticides are also used indoors, to spray for roaches, for example, and these pesticides can often cause an allergic reaction.

NATURAL MEDICINE AND INORGANIC ALLERGIES

Natural medicine is an excellent antidote for the ills caused by modern civilization. Chemicals and pollutants interfere with our natural ability to stay healthy, resulting in conditions like allergic reaction. Natural medicine alternatives, on the other hand, restore the connection among mind, body, and spirit, and help the body to heal itself. Natural medicine can be helpful both in treating the symptoms of inorganic allergy as well as in rejuvenating the body's natural healing abilities.

Inorganic allergies can result in some of the same symptoms as those caused by other allergies, such as hay fever and food allergy. While treatments for these symptoms are included in this chapter, you may also want to refer to other chapters for additional suggestions for relieving your specific symptoms. Stress is a major factor in inorganic allergy, and stress reductions are emphasized among the alternatives discussed in this chapter.

Acupressure

Acupressure, described in more depth in Chapter 3, can be applied to relieve the symptoms of inorganic allergy. These symptoms include those described under the acupressure heading in other chapters.

While inorganic allergies can result in a wide range of symptoms, here are some acupressure techniques for relieving some of the more common ones:

Headache Acupressure is an excellent means of ridding yourself of headaches. Depending on the location of your headache, points are selected distally to release your headaches. For example, for headaches at the temples, use

point TW 5. For headaches along the forehead, use point
LI 4. For headaches at the top of your head, you may use
point LI 20. (See diagrams on pages 384 through 387.)
Acupressure practitioners reduce headache through points
near the bridge of the nose and the back of the skull. Tilt
your head back, and with your right thumb, press the
point in the center of the base of the skull. With your left
thumb and index finger, press in the upper hollows of the
eye socket near the bridge of the nose. Breathe deeply for
a couple of minutes.

Headache and Indigestion   Another way of relieving
a headache as well as indigestion is through a point between the eyebrows, referred to as the Third Eye point
(Yingtang). Hold your palms together, and tilt your head
downward. Place your index and middle fingers of both
hands between your eyebrows, in the indentation where
the bridge of the nose meets the forehead. Focus your
mind on this spot and breathe deeply while pressing. Hold
the position for at least two minutes. Also, use point LI 4
for headaches with indigestion.

Frontal Headache   Headache pain located at the
front of your head can be relieved by pressing a point on
the webbing between the thumb and index finger (point
LI 4). Place your right hand over the top of your left hand.
With your thumb, press the webbing between the thumb
and index finger of your left hand. Press toward that bone
connecting with the index finger. Hold this for at least one
minute, while breathing slowly and deeply, and then repeat the exercise on the other hand.

Affirmations

Environmental pollutants as well as psychological stress place your immune system on alert, and it becomes oversensitive. You probably make the situation even worse by giving yourself verbal messages about how stressed out you are, how on edge you feel. Maybe you look out at the smog in the air or pass the smokestack of a factory, and say something like "I'm in trouble now." These are called negative affirmations, and if you say them often enough, with conviction, your immune system takes you at your word and reacts accordingly, most likely with some allergy symptoms. Even if you aren't necessarily conscious of these messages, chances are you're expecting the worst.

On the other hand, positive affirmations have the opposite effect on your immune system. You can use them to calm yourself, and send messages of relaxation and well-being that, in turn, relieve the edginess and hypersensitivity that results in allergic reaction.

Here are a few affirmations to use for relieving the stress that can result in inorganic allergic reactions:

- I am safe in my home and community. I can relax and let go of the fear and stress that I've been holding inside.

- I am breathing in calm and pure air, and exhaling all of the toxins that have built up inside of me. Nature is cleaning out my system.

- I accept life's challenges and become stronger every day.

Think about the chemicals and other pollutants that affect you the most and make up affirmations that counteract their effects on you. Write them on paper or on small cards and keep them handy as reminders of positive self-talk. You may even want to tape them up over your kitchen sink or near the bathroom mirror to keep yourself focused.

The best time to say affirmations is during the morning, when your mind is fresh, as well as in the evening before bedtime. You may also want to record your affirmations on tape and then play it when you're driving, or working around the house.

Aromatherapy

Aromatherapy can be highly useful in treating the effects of inorganic allergies and chronic industrial irritants. First of all, the essential oils help to promote general good health, peace of mind, and the ability to withstand the pressures of daily life. And aromatherapy can be applied in treating the effects of the industrial irritants as they affect the skin, respiratory system, and gastrointestinal system.

The essential oils of aromatherapy, some of which are described in more detail in Chapter 4, affect subconscious parts of your mind that cause a release of positive energy that helps to counteract whatever symptoms you may be experiencing. A qualified aromatherapist will listen as you discuss your symptoms and will also ask you questions about your household and your normal routine. He or she will then make recommendations about the essential oils that might be most helpful, and how and when to use them.

Because we are chronically exposed to many industrial irritants through the atmosphere, using essential oils in an aroma lamp will be a standard part of your treatment. You may also be instructed to inhale an essential oil from a bowl of steaming hot water. Other oils will be applied directly to the skin, particularly in treating skin irritations. Other oils may be ingested, though you are not advised to do this without consulting a qualified aromatherapist and your physician.

A range of essential oils is useful in relieving the effects of inorganic allergies. A few of these essential oils are discussed below.

Breathing Difficulties and Coughing   The essential oil of the cedar tree, particularly those grown in Morocco and Algeria, offers lifegiving and calming effects. Cedar oil also has beneficial effects on the bronchial system and is a good expectorant that helps to relieve coughing. Place a few drops of cedar oil in an aroma lamp. If desired, cedar can be mixed with lemon or hyssop.

The oil of the cypress tree acts in harmony with the central nervous system, bringing serenity and strengthening connective tissues. Cypress is known to stop excess flow and as such is an excellent expectorant that relieves lung congestion. Place a few drops of cypress oil in an aroma lamp, or obtain a salve from your aromatherapist that includes cypress oil and rub it directly on the back and chest.

The healing powers of eucalyptus have been, and continue to be, widely known as a treatment for respiratory difficulties. In fact, many cough medications available in your drugstore contain eucalyptus, as do various topical preparations for treating pain. The whole breathing process is actually aided by eucalyptus, because it helps to regenerate lung tissue as well as acting as an expectorant and decongestant. Place a few drops of eucalyptus in an aroma lamp for relief of coughing and wheezing. You may also want to talk to your aromatherapist about obtaining a natural ointment that you can rub into your chest at night.

Of all the essential oils used in the practice of aromatherapy, rosemary is among the most common. Rosemary is believed to strengthen, and promote awareness, because of its effect on the central nervous system. As such, it is especially useful in conjunction with meditation and visualization. For treating general respiratory symptoms, place a few drops of rosemary essential oil in an aroma lamp. Rosemary may also be taken internally but, as always, check with an aromatherapist first.

Skin Irritation Chamomile is associated with relaxation and the promotion of well-being and is often consumed as an herbal tea. The essential oil of chamomile has these same properties, and it is useful in treating conditions related to nervousness and anxiety, including both stomach and skin disorders. Chamomile can lessen the symptoms of eczema, hives, and rashes. A few drops can be added to bathwater, it can be used in a massage oil, and a few drops can be applied to the affected areas in a diluted form. Additionally, a few drops can be added to an aroma lamp. Consult an aromatherapist before taking chamomile internally.

Immortelle oil is noted for helping people to look within themselves and achieve awareness. It also has a history of being used as a treatment for disorders of the skin, lymphatic system, and mucous membranes, particularly disorders resulting from irritants in the environment. Immortelle is helpful for treating allergy-related rashes, often in conjunction with lavender and rockrose. Immortelle can be used in an aroma lamp in a bath, or in a base oil (with the assistance of an aromatherapist).

Gastrointestinal Problems One of the major uses of chamomile oil is in relieving the symptoms of stomach and intestinal problems. Place a few drops in an aroma lamp or in a warm bath, and breathe in its calming and healing aroma. You can also obtain relief from extreme cramps by soaking a compress in hot water with a few drops of chamomile added to it. Make sure the water is comfortably but not excessively hot. Soak the compress again in the water and reapply it.

Aromatherapy can be useful in conjunction with meditation and yoga by helping to create a calming and health-promoting environment. If symptoms persist, get in contact with a physician. Do this immediately if breathing becomes difficult or if symptoms become otherwise life threatening.

Botanical Medicine

The philosophy of botanical medicine makes it a great complementary treatment for inorganic allergies. To understand the reason for this complementary relationship start with the cause of this form of allergy. Inorganic allergies are caused primarily by the environment, including the chemicals and industrial irritants that constantly impinge upon us. And think back to Chapter 3 to the philosophy of many botanical medicine practitioners. The herbs that are most effective are those that are available in our geographical region. Inorganic allergies are caused by our environment, and botanical medicine relies on this same environment, using herbs that harness the healing energy around you to effect a treatment.

Botanical medicine can be useful in treating the symptoms that result from reactions to chemical irritants. For example, herbs can be used to treat red, itchy eyes, difficulty in breathing, skin irritations, and stomach problems. Some of these remedies will be described later in this section. However, the real strength of botanical medicine in treating inorganic allergies lies in the usefulness of herbs in strengthening and rejuvenating the various organs and systems of the human body. By focusing on building strength and vitality, you build up your overall ability to maintain internal balance and enhanced energy, in spite of your environment.

To treat inorganic allergies with botanical medicine, focus first on prevention—regulating your metabolism and the balance of fluids, building up resistance to disease, and increasing energy. Herbal teas used on a daily basis, supplemented by tonics, will be useful in keeping your internal systems operating at their peak. Pay close attention to the symptoms you suffer from most, respiratory or gastrointestinal, for example, and select herbs that specifically address the needs of these systems. Also consider using herbal-based emollients and oils that will make your skin more supple and healthy, and less susceptible to eruptions of hives, eczema, or other rashes.

Environmentalists often tell us that we are the victims of a sick environment. Through botanical medicine, we can seek out and make use of the healing elements in our environment. Here are some preparations that you can use to build up your resistance to industrial pollutants.

Improving and Strengthening Circulation Soaking in a bath of gingerroot will stimulate circulation as well as provide an overall warming effect on the body. Make a ginger tea, using the recipe from Chapter 4, in great enough quantities to be able fill your bathtub with one-third ginger tea and two-thirds water. Make the water as hot as you can tolerate without being uncomfortable. Relax and soak as the ginger strengthens your circulation system and enhances your ability to stand up to the pollutants in your environment.

When used in a compress, ginger not only enhances your circulation but also increases your energy, builds up your immune system, and helps to cut down on the accumulation of toxins in your body. Here's how to make a ginger compress:

1. Make a strong ginger tea.
2. Drop a washcloth into the tea and let it soak for ten minutes.
3. Lift the washcloth out of the tea by using tongs, and wring it out quickly.
4. Place the washcloth on your chest, your lower back, or any other area you want to warm and stimulate.
5. Cover the washcloth with a towel and, if possible, place a hot water bottle on top of that to hold in the warmth.
6. Relax in a comfortable position and leave it in place for up to a half hour.

Chest Congestion and Coughing   The chest congestion or coughing that often results from exposure to environmental pollutants can be relieved by rubbing a small amount of eucalyptus oil directly into your chest. This can be done before bed to allow the healing action to occur as you sleep.

You can also treat coughing with a mixture of herbal oils, which you can purchase at a health food store. Mix an ounce each of the herbal oils of cinnamon, eucalyptus, thyme, camphor, and marjoram. Add a few drops of olive oil to dilute this mixture, and store it in a bottle. Spread it on your chest at bedtime—it will have a healing and soothing action that will help relieve cough and congestion, while enhancing the vitality of your respiratory system.

Skin Irritations   The herb derived from the roots and seeds of the burdock plant is especially useful in treating skin irritations. Burdock is an excellent cleanser of the blood and the lymphatic system, and has been used with much success in clearing up various kinds of rashes. Burdock also contains iron, so when taken internally, it strengthens the blood and, because it detoxifies the liver, it also has a relaxing effect. When using burdock to treat skin conditions, it is best applied externally as an oil. While you can purchase burdock oil from a health food store, or from a practitioner, the following are directions for creating your own supply:

1. Mash approximately two ounces of burdock herb in your hands, and place it in a glass jar.
2. Add two ounces of either olive or sesame oil and seal the jar.
3. Shake the sealed jar every day for two weeks.
4. Strain the contents through a cheesecloth to remove the herb fragments.
5. Pour this mixture into a clean jar, add some vitamin E to help preserve the contents, and seal the jar.

Rub the burdock oil on the affected areas at least once per day until the symptoms have subsided.

Skin irritations can also be treated with the use of the marshmallow herb, which is derived from the roots of the plant. When used in tea, marshmallow acts as a tonic to strengthen the body and enhance internal vitality. This can help fortify you against the toxins that can lead to allergic reaction and skin problems. Marshmallow can either be used externally in a poultice to treat skin eruptions or drunk as a tea.

To make a tea with marshmallow, follow these steps:

1. Place one ounce of marshmallow herb in a pint of water.

2. Heat the water until it boils.

3. Bring the water down to a simmer, and continue to heat for sixty minutes.

4. Strain the tea into a cup.

Drink three cups per day of marshmallow herb tea, and feel its soothing and revitalizing effects.

To use marshmallow herb in a poultice, follow these steps:

1. Crumble a few grams of marshmallow herb using a mortar and pestle or small blender.

2. Add enough hot water to form a paste.

3. Rub the paste on the affected area, and then either cover it with a cloth, or wrap a bandage on it. Leave it on a few hours, and then replace it with a fresh poultice until the symptoms are healed. If you experience an adverse reaction, discontinue use.

Gastrointestinal Complaints Aniseed is a warm herb, useful in treating the stomach, liver, and kidneys. You probably have a supply of anise on your spice rack, and are familiar with its spicy taste. Anise warms the digestive system and whole abdominal area, and relieves nausea and gas, reduces abdominal pains, and stimulates digestion. The easiest way to administer anise is in a hot cup of tea, using the following directions:

1. Crush one teaspoonful of aniseed either by using a mortar and pestle or by taking the rounded side of a spoon and mashing the herb in a small bowl.
2. Bring one pint of water to a boil.
3. Remove the water from direct heat, and drop in the aniseed.
4. Let it steep for a few minutes, covered, and then remove the aniseed, using a fine-mesh tea strainer or cheesecloth.

You can drink three cups or more of anise tea each day, or as needed to treat your symptoms. You may also want to make a great-tasting tea that includes not only anise but also ginger, cinnamon, and cardamom. Make it a habit of having a cup of this tea after each meal to promote digestion. As an aftermeal tea, fennel can be used for similar results.

Cayenne is another commonly used herb, both in the kitchen as well as in the creation of herbal treatments. Cayenne is a hot herb, known for its stimulating effect on blood circulation and digestion. It is also used in treating cramps and diarrhea, as an appetite stimulant, and for help in dispelling gas. Cayenne has such a beneficial effect on the stomach, even though it is spicy, that in small doses, it is even useful for clearing up stomach ulcers.

Administer cayenne by dropping a pinch of cayenne powder into a glass of water, and then stirring it vigorously to mix it. Even if you like cayenne on your food, your taste buds will need some time in getting used to the unadorned flavor of cayenne. Initially, keep the amount you use small, and gradually build it up to experience the full benefits. If the cayenne causes you to feel a wave of nausea, don't worry about it because it should pass quickly and you will begin to experience a relief of your other symptoms. While cayenne is a safe herb, use it cautiously. If you find it is irritating your stomach, discontinue use.

Try some of these botanical remedies and see how they work for you. You may want to combine botanical medicine with meditation and allow the two approaches to work together in helping you to relax and rejuvenate.

Holistic Massage

At times, the chemicals and other pollutants in your environment can seem to conspire against you, compounded by noise and just plain negative energy from the fast-paced world we live in. Holistic massage helps bring your system back into balance, restoring feelings of calm and relaxation, so that you are more in control of your feelings and reactions.

Holistic massage is described in Chapter 4, and you may want to review this section. Try scheduling a weekly massage, either with a practitioner or with your partner. It will promote your sense of connection with other people, and dispel the sense of alienation that can keep you on edge and hypersensitive. If you do practice massage with a partner, work out your own strokes by telling each other what feels good. You'll not only get a massage that really works for you but also promote communication and mutual trust.

As you practice massage, keep in mind that the parts of your body work together as a whole, and it is important to focus your efforts on all parts of the body, from the head to the feet, to promote a state of complete relaxation. Massage works well with other relaxation techniques, including meditation.

Homeopathy

The chemicals and other pollutants in the environment and the additives in food can create imbalances in your system that make your body sick as it attempts to fight off the toxicity. Homeopathy treats inorganic allergy in the same way as other forms of allergy—as signs that the body's natural defenses need a stimulus to help it complete the healing cycle. Thus, homeopathy treats both the symptoms associated with allergies that result from chemical irritants and helps to maintain system balance and vitality.

If the reactions you are having to toxins in your environment are relatively predictable, and are causing noticeable discomfort, it is advisable to talk with a homeopathic physician about undergoing a treatment program. A range of homeopathic remedies may be helpful with inorganic allergies, depending on your constitution, and these medicines will not add chemicals to your system that simply mask symptoms, as would many conventional medicines. Your homeopathic practitioner will most likely also recommend that you avoid allergens wherever possible, particularly when you are reacting to household items that can be eliminated.

Here are some homeopathic remedies that may help with specific symptoms related to inorganic allergies. You should check with your doctor before taking any remedy to make sure it is appropriate for you.

Headache   One of the most commonly used homeopathic medicines for headache is belladonna, derived from deadly nightshade. Headache symptoms compatible with the use of this remedy include intense pain, with sensitivity to noise and light and other stimuli around you. This pain probably comes on rapidly, and is usually focused in the forehead. The face may be hot while the hands and feet are cold.

Other headache remedies include Nux vomica for headaches that are accompanied by irritability and often occur after overeating, or drinking coffee or alcohol. Pulsatilla, on the other hand, is often associated with digestive upset. Take one dose up to every two hours, for a total of three doses, and discontinue it when symptoms get better. If three doses do not help, try another medicine.

Congestion and Coughing   Environmental pollution that results in allergy symptoms such as nasal congestion and coughing can be relieved by Wyethia. Wyethia may benefit you if your symptoms include an intense itching sensation on the soft palate of your mouth or itching behind your nose. Symptoms may also include a dry feeling in your throat and nasal passages, even though your nose is running.

Arsenicum album, which is derived from arsenic trioxide, may be a useful medicine if your allergies also include wheezing. Arsenicum is generally used as a cold medication. Symptoms that indicate a need for arsenicum include violent sneezing, a strong burning sensation in the nasal passages, headache, coughing, and constricted air passages with some wheezing. Other indications of the need for arsenicum include experiencing some relief from coughing after drinking warm liquid, and a burning sensation in the chest.

When using any of these medicines, first try one dose and wait for a reaction. Generally, you will be provided with dosage information by your homeopathic medicine supplier, or the standard dose will be indicated on the container. If taking a dose of the medicine causes your symptoms to improve, wait until the symptoms return before you take any more. If your symptoms do not improve

after four hours, take another dose and wait another few
hours before considering a different remedy.

Gastrointestinal Complaints Arsenicum is also one
of the more commonly used homeopathic medicines for
treating ailments of the gastrointestinal system with symptoms that include vomiting, diarrhea, and stomach or intestinal pain.

Ipecac is a useful homeopathic medicine if the major
symptom is nausea, with or without diarrhea or vomiting.
Ipecac is used by individuals who are most likely not as
seriously ill as those needing arsenicum. Nausea continues, even after vomiting, and it is made worse even by the
smell of food. Some diarrhea and gas may accompany the
nausea.

Generally, these medicines should be given once per
hour until the symptoms begin to subside. When using a
homeopathic medicine for possible food allergy symptoms,
you should notice improvements rather quickly. If not,
switch to another homeopathic medicine. And again, if
symptoms become severe, get medical assistance.

Skin Irritations Contact dermatitis commonly results from touching a household chemical like a cleaning
fluid. Rhus toxicodendron, derived from poison ivy, is a
useful treatment for symptoms that include burning, itching, and fluid-filled skin eruptions that seem to be worse at
night, in open air, and while lying in a warm bed. The
itching may also worsen after scratching, which may be
relieved after immersion in very hot water. Feelings of
restlessness and irritability are also clues that Rhus toxicodendron might be a good match with this set of symptoms.

An allergic reaction in which the skin is inflamed and
blistered, but not itching, might call for croton oil. A rash

requiring croton oil is also itchy, and might first be relieved by scratching it a bit. However, this action causes
the rash to become so inflamed that even touching it
lightly causes pain. Additionally, a rash treatable by croton
oil will usually be worse around the eyes, on the scalp and
in the genital area.

Other homeopathic remedies are also useful in treating
contact dermatitis, with each prescription based on differences in the appearance and associated symptoms of this
ailment. Bryonia, for example, is prescribed for a rash that
includes dry bumps, accompanied by feelings of irritability. Anacardium is used when symptoms include blisters
filled with a yellow fluid.

If you are not currently under the care of a medical
doctor, homeopathy can be useful in helping you to build
up your system to withstand the effects of the irritants in
our environment. Homeopathy is also beneficial when
combined with breathing exercises to strengthen your
lungs. Meditation and massage will help you to attain the
serenity needed to maintain your center and stay relaxed.
If your symptoms are of such a severity that you are being
treated by a physician, let him or her know that you are
also using homeopathic remedies.

Naturopathy

Treatment of inorganic allergies, and the effects of exposure to alien substances like chronic industrial irritants are
a natural match with the philosophy and techniques of
naturopathy. Supporting and rebuilding the immune system, for example, is a hallmark of naturopathic practice,
and practitioners use a range of diets and herbal preparations to keep the immune system working at its peak. The
liver plays an important role here as the organ responsible

for detoxifying the harmful chemicals with which the body is constantly bombarded. And because naturopaths view the body, mind, and emotions as working together in determining our overall state of health, the effects of stress, and ways to cope with it, are also a concern of naturopaths.

Naturopathy presents a realm of possibilities for building up your stamina for coping with the chemical and emotional stresses of modern life. While you will need to work with a naturopath in establishing your own individualized wellness program, some of the options are outlined below.

Enhancing Your Immune System Toxins can weaken your immune system and make you more vulnerable, so that all sorts of bacteria and allergens, as well as many household chemicals, can lead to major allergic reactions. The operation of the thymus, the major gland in the immune system, can become weakened by factors like a poor diet or too much stress. The thymus produces T cells, which are white blood cells that play a role in immunity and help protect you from viruses and infections, and are also involved in preventing allergy. With stress and environmental toxins depleting the energy of the thymus gland, you're at a distinct disadvantage when new toxins find their way into your environment.

Naturopaths treat thymus gland deficiencies with vitamin supplements. Vitamins C and E, as well as selenium and zinc, provide needed nutrients to enhance the function of the thymus. Naturopaths also use herbal medicines in treating immune system deficiencies. Echinacea and licorice, for example, have been shown to have a positive effect on the thymus gland. As the thymus is strengthened, you are better able to withstand the pollutants around you.

Naturopaths also focus on other parts of the immune system in helping to build you up against the effects of toxic chemicals. The lymphatic system, which is involved in keeping your system cleansed of bacteria and cell debris and fighting illness, can be strengthened through a range of techniques. Exercise and deep breathing, for example, increase the circulation of lymph throughout your body. Herbs like echinacea and goldenseal, as well as ginseng, stimulate lymph function. The flow of blood through the spleen, the largest organ in the lymph system, is enhanced by goldenseal.

Other aspects of the immune system include white blood cells, which include lymphocytes, or T cells, and monocytes, all of which are involved in cleansing the system of toxins and fighting off bacteria. Naturopaths also use herbal medicines, particularly echinacea, in enhancing the function of the white blood cells.

Naturopaths view stress as being an important factor in how we physically react to our environment. Stress causes the adrenal gland to increase the production of hormones that inhibit white blood cell production and cause the thymus to shrink. As a result, the immune system is suppressed and you become much more susceptible to disease. Recommended treatments for stress include meditation and visualization, as well as rest and relaxation.

Naturopaths also treat the immune system with nutrition, through a diet that includes adequate protein and low amounts of sugar and fat.

Supporting the Liver Naturopathic treatment for inorganic allergies generally includes support for enhanced liver function. When you are exposed to toxins, it is your liver that bears most of the burden. For example, all of the toxins you eat in your food, including pesticides and preservatives, are detoxified by the liver. It secretes bile, which helps you to absorb fat-soluble substances, including vitamins. The liver is also involved in storing vitamins and minerals and the production of histamine, which results in allergies.

Naturopaths view the liver as playing a major role in the development of allergies. When it is constantly exposed to toxic chemicals, as well as drugs and alcohol, it becomes sluggish, and its ability to do its job of detoxification is impaired. The result is sensitivity to chemicals and industrial irritants.

The naturopathic approach to enhancing the functioning of the liver is, as always, holistic. It begins with diet, eliminating saturated fats that cause the liver to become fatty and sluggish. Dietary fiber, on the other hand, promotes secretion of bile. Organically grown foods, as free as possible from pesticides and other chemicals, are recommended. Vitamin C and E, as well as zinc and selenium, help to protect the liver from being damaged from the chemicals that pass through it. Fatty liver is also prevented by eating legumes and egg yolk.

Botanical medicines are also useful in enhancing the detoxification capabilities of the liver. Dandelion root enhances the production and flow of bile and improves overall liver function. Milk thistle also protects the liver against damage from the toxins that pass through it daily, as do artichoke leaves.

Reducing Stress   Reducing stress greatly enhances the body's strength. As briefly discussed earlier in this section, there is a physical reason for this. When you feel stressed, the adrenal glands secrete hormones to maintain the balance of many functions like heart rate and digestion. Over time, repeated stress may exhaust the adrenal glands. As a result, you are more prone to allergic reaction, asthma, high blood pressure, immune suppression, and a range of other conditions.

Naturopaths recommend lifestyle changes, diet, nutritional supplements, and botanical preparations as a means of reducing stress and its negative effects on health. Exercise is viewed as a stress reducer. A regular exercise program can enhance your self-esteem and help you feel more in control of your life. Exercise also improves your endurance and energy and strengthens your heart and respiratory system, while reducing your heart rate and blood pressure. It also reduces the overproduction of your adrenal glands in reaction to stressful situations.

Naturopaths also recommend relaxation exercises to help keep you in a more positive frame of mind. Relaxation can involve getting more rest and sleep and taking time out for enjoyable activities like reading and watching television. A naturopath might also recommend relaxation tapes for you to listen to, to teach yourself how to create a state of relaxation. Visualization and meditation might also be recommended.

Because the health of your adrenal glands is important in resisting the effects of environmental toxins, naturopaths also recommend the use of herbs and nutritional supplements in supporting the functions of the adrenals. Potassium strengthens the adrenals, and potassium can be obtained by eating foods like avocado, lima beans, bananas, peaches, white meat chicken, lamb, and cod.

Nutrients needed to support the manufacture of hormones by the adrenal glands include vitamins C and B_6, zinc, and magnesium. These nutrients are included in many multivitamin and mineral formulas, and are especially important during periods of high stress. Pantothenic acid is another nutrient important to the adrenal glands, and while it can be obtained through nutritional supplements, it is also present in whole grains and legumes, veg-

etables like broccoli and cauliflower, salmon and liver, and
other foods.

The Chinese herb, ginseng, has a long history of use in
strengthening the functioning of the adrenal glands. Ginseng is useful in periods of stress, and helps protect you
from physical and mental fatigue. Ginseng acts directly on
the nervous system to help you keep calm during moments of stress, and is also good protection against environmental toxins, as well as the effects of noise, heat,
heavy work loads, and other stresses of daily life. A dose of
one or two grams of ginseng per day is recommended to
provide you with a constant supply of the balancing and
adrenal-enhancing effects of ginseng.

Working with a Naturopath   Going to a naturopath
can be a great place to start in creating a healthier lifestyle and preventing environmentally caused allergic reactions. Your naturopath will begin by asking you a lot of
questions about what you eat, what your current emotional state is like, and the kinds of symptoms you are
having and when. He or she will also most likely give you
some kind of examination to look for symptoms that indicate imbalances that are leaving you vulnerable. Expect
your naturopath to take a holistic approach to your condition, with recommendations for lifestyle changes, including diet and exercise, perhaps supplemented by vitamins
and herbal tonics and remedies. He or she will draw on
nutrition, homeopathy, and botanical medicine, as well as
meditation, counseling, visualization, and other practices.

Naturopathy can make all the difference in empower-
ing you to take more control over your health. However,
keep a close eye on your own symptoms. If you find that
your allergy symptoms interfere with your ability to accomplish what you need to do every day, or if they become debilitating at times, consider seeing a medical doc-

tor. This is especially true if you have difficulty breathing at times.

Meditation

Meditation is a great way to relax when faced with the stresses of daily life. And when you feel an allergic reaction coming on, or are in the midst of one, creating a sense of peace and relaxation will also calm the immune system. Scientific evidence supports this theory, as research has shown that meditation can lower blood pressure as well as heart and respiratory rates.

The best approach to meditation is to learn a technique and then practice it on a daily basis, even if it is for only a few minutes every day, generally in the morning. The result of this practice is a sense of calm that will stay with you during the remainder of the day. Additionally, with practice you will be able to use your meditation technique to help achieve calm when you suddenly find yourself in a stressful situation, especially one in which you might be more susceptible to allergens.

A technique for meditating is presented in Chapter 4.

Reflexology

Reflexology is useful for keeping the energy balanced among your vital organs, and promoting relaxation, so that you are better able to withstand the toxins in your environment, and maintain a centered, relaxed composure. Because reflexology is generally practiced in partnership with another person, it also promotes a sense of connectedness with others—certainly something we are often missing in our fast-paced lives. Reflexology is described in Chapters 3 and 6.

The Lungs You have a lung reflex area on both your hands and your feet. For a description of how reflexology can work to strengthen your lungs, refer to pp. 240–241.

The Kidneys The kidneys are responsible for filtering toxic substances out of your blood, and keeping the fluid balances in the tissues regulated. When the kidneys are out of balance, toxins can build up in your system to the point that you experience allergic reactions. The reflex areas that correspond with the kidneys are located on the hands and feet. This area is on the palms of the hands, inside of the tendon to the thumb, just below the index finger. On the feet, the kidney reflex area is in the middle of the arch, almost at the center of the sole.

To apply reflexology to the hand, locate the kidney reflex area and press it with the thumb of the other hand. Press it lightly the first time, release it slightly, then press again, this time a bit more firmly. Repeat this action seven times, increasing the pressure each time.

To apply reflexology to the feet, locate the kidney reflex area in the arch of your foot on the sole and press it with the thumb of your other hand. Use the same technique as you did with your hand, pressing lightly, releasing, then pressing more firmly. Do this seven times, gradually increasing the pressure.

Remember that you have two kidneys. Massage both feet and both hands.

The Stomach One of the first places that stress shows up is in the stomach, with symptoms of nausea, cramps, tightness. To make matters worse, when we consume food additives and other toxins, they hit the stomach full force. Reflexology techniques focused on the stomach help it to work more efficiently. In turn, the stomach is less likely to go into a reactive mode as different foods are introduced. Additionally, if the stomach is working smoothly, recovery from an allergic reaction will be more complete.

The reflex points for the stomach are located on both hands and feet, though because the stomach is located off-center, toward the right side of the body, the stomach reflex areas are larger on the left hand and left foot. The stomach reflex area on the left hand is located on the palm, right under the pads below the ring finger, middle finger, and index finger. It is a smaller area on the right palm, just below the index finger. The stomach reflex area on the left foot is on the sole, almost halfway down, between the toes and the heel. It extends from the big toe to the fourth toe. It is in the same position on the right foot, but is located only under the big toe.

When working the stomach reflex area on the left hand, use your thumb to massage the whole area in a circular motion. Start under the ring finger and move toward the index finger, pressing lightly the first time, and then pressing slightly harder each time, for a total of seven repetitions. Repeat the same motions on the right hand, but only under the index finger.

When massaging the left foot, use the same circular massage technique as you used on the left hand, starting under the big toe and moving outward toward the fourth toe. Repeat this outward massage movement seven times, slightly increasing the pressure each time. Also perform this massage on your right foot, but only in the area under your big toe.

When you try these exercises, don't forget to regulate your breathing. Inhale as you press with your thumb, and exhale as you release the pressure.

Applying Reflexology

As you do reflexology exercises, visualize yourself in a
healthy and calm environment, like the beach or a forest,
breathing fresh, clean air. Imagine that you are breathing
out all the toxins trapped inside your body.

Visualization

No matter where you live—in the country or in an urban
setting—you are exposed to air pollution, harmful substances from the food you eat, noise, and emotional stress.
Visualization, described in more depth in Chapter 3, can
help you to surround yourself with an atmosphere of calm
and serenity. Visualization works from the inside out, and
when you visualize the kind of environment you want to
live in, one that promotes health and well-being, you begin to experience the feelings that accompany that kind of
environment. And with practice you can maintain this serenity regardless of what happens around you.

Here is a visualization to help you remain calm and
centered in a world of allergens and industrial irritants.

Find a quiet place, where you can sit alone for a while.
Sit in an upright position or lie flat on your back, whatever
is more comfortable. You may want to play some quiet
music in the background.

Imagine your body as an overwhelming, dirty, dangerous city.

Now imagine a sense of peace and calm overtaking the
city. The air is clear. There is a blue sky. The sun is shining at every corner. People on the streets are relaxed and
smile at each other.

Your immune system is alert but relaxed. The real dan-
ger is gone.

Remain relaxed and focus your concentration on the

feelings of relaxation and security that are now flowing throughout your "inner city." Think of how the city looks so bright and clean. Breathe in the pure air, and exhale slowly. Feel the sunlight on your skin. Enjoy the trust you have in those around you.

You may want to modify this visualization to fit your own living circumstances, picturing your own community and putting real faces on the people walking the streets. Try this visualization often, even every few days, especially when you are experiencing stress.

It takes years of practice to create the negative images we all carry around, and counteracting them with positive images will take time and practice. Don't be surprised if you are uncomfortable with the process at first, and even unable to create a visualization. Focus on learning to relax, then begin imagining situations from your past in which you felt secure and happy. Once you teach yourself to relax and create positive visualizations, you can begin targeting your visualizations toward new situations you want to create in your life.

Yoga

Yoga is an excellent practice for promoting relaxation and keeping your lungs, as well as the rest of your body, exercised and healthy. Hatha yoga stresses the importance of body and mind awareness and teaches various deep, lung-expanding breathing and relaxation techniques to achieve this awareness. To learn more about yoga and to try a basic breathing exercise, see pages 244–245.

CHAPTER NINE

Skin Allergies and Eczema

Skin allergy is a broad term that covers a wide range of symptoms with an even wider range of potential triggers. While skin allergy has its roots in the immune system, much like other forms of allergy, symptoms can be caused by contact with an allergen, a change in temperature, or may be the result of emotion, to name a few of the possible triggers.

Chapter 9 focuses on three forms of skin allergy—allergic dermatitis, hives, and eczema—and what you can do to get relief.

Contact Dermatitis

Have you ever put on a new shirt right out of the box and broken out in what looked like hives? The cause was most likely contact dermatitis. Contact dermatitis, as the name implies, is the result of touching an allergenic substance. What is unique about contact dermatitis is that it is the result of prolonged interaction with the offending substance, as you would experience from wearing a shirt for a period of time. Also, the symptoms of contact dermatitis are localized to wherever the interaction occurs, rather than all over the body. So if the shirt was causing the reaction, the rash would appear on the chest, neck and arms.

While any number of substances can result in a reaction for contact dermatitis sufferers, here is a list of some of the common ones.

Forehead	hatbands, hair dye
Back of the neck	hair dye
Eyelids	cosmetics
Earlobes	earrings
Face	cosmetics, shaving lotion, aftershave, shaving cream
Bridge of the nose	glasses
Armpits	deodorant, clothing
Nose	soap, cosmetics, or toiletries
Feet	socks, shoes made of synthetic materials
Hands	chemicals, metal, rubber, plants, household detergents
Legs	clothing

The substances most likely to result in an allergic dermatitis reaction include cosmetics, metal, clothing, plants, and rubber.

Hives

Hives are also referred to as urticaria. The symptoms of hives include welts—small, red, round, and swollen areas of the skin that are generally itchy. These swollen areas may be large, from the beginning, or because small swollen areas have gradually spread into other swollen areas. Hives can also be accompanied by swelling of certain body parts, like the tongue, lips, hands, and feet. A case of hives may be acute, meaning that it can last from a few hours to a few weeks. Others suffer from chronic hives that last far longer than a few weeks. The welts caused by hives may appear in one place on the body and then disappear after a short period of time, only to appear at a different spot later. Scratching makes them much worse.

Like other allergies, hives are caused by an overproduction of histamine in the skin and the tissues just below the skin. This histamine dilates the walls of blood vessels, allowing fluids to leak out into the surrounding tissues. Itching and swelling result. However, the reason for the production of this histamine is very hard to pinpoint. For example, exposure to sunlight or to a sun lamp can cause hives. Extreme cold can also be a trigger, as can drinking cold liquids. And an even more common cause of hives is drugs such as tetracycline, penicillin, sulfa, phenobarbital, aspirin, and tranquilizers. Food allergy is yet another culprit (discussed in Chapter 10). Foods that commonly cause hives include nuts, tomatoes, shellfish, and berries. Additionally, wearing a constricting belt or tight clothes or rubbing with a towel can cause hives.

A condition that often accompanies hives, called angioedema, can cause swelling in the deeper layers of the skin, including the hands, feet, and face. It can also occur in the throat, and this swelling can interfere with the ability to breathe or swallow. This can be a life-threatening situation and when it happens, emergency treatment is needed.

Hives can also be strongly influenced by the emotions. Feelings of fear, depression, panic, anxiety . . . these can all result in a case of hives.

Allergic Eczema

The symptoms of allergic eczema, also referred to as atopic dermatitis, are dry and itching skin. Allergic eczema can occur in infants as well as children and adults. In infants, eczema is often associated with an allergy to foods such as milk, eggs, cereal, and some fruits and vegetables. This relationship between allergic eczema and food is not so strong in older children and adults.

Allergic eczema results in the appearance of skin lesions or patches on the skin that are dry and cracked or scaly. These patches are usually found in creases of the body, including areas of the wrist and forearm, around the eyes and ears, on the face and neck, behind the ears and knees. Again, the main symptom of allergic eczema is itching. This itching can be the start of a vicious circle because most people respond by scratching, which results in redness of the skin and more itching. Eczema can spread from one area of your body to others, with lesions that swell and ooze.

Emotional Aspects of Skin Allergies

If you are an allergic dermatitis or eczema sufferer, you have probably noticed that your reactions are more severe at some times than others. Your emotional state has a large effect on how often your skin allergies flare up, and with what level of severity.

Anger, if it is not discussed and resolved, or otherwise released, for example, through yelling or pounding a pillow, can stay inside and intensify. This unreleased anger can manifest itself on your hands or other parts of your body if you have a tendency toward skin allergies. You might find yourself taking out your anger on yourself, digging at your hands or arms, unconsciously or even in your sleep. This reaction is so pronounced in some individuals that they have scratched bald spots on their scalp.

When you have turned your anger inward on yourself, rather than dealing with the source of the anger, any tendency toward skin allergy can provide you with an all-too-easy target. Itching and digging at your skin can cause damage, even serious damage, and this is self-destructive behavior.

While emotions are not the whole picture, they can help to trigger a skin allergy as well as cause the reaction to be more severe.

Spiritual Aspects of Skin Allergy

Continuing our own unique spiritual growth and development requires change, and change is something that all of us fear to some extent. If your fear of change is so strong that it keeps you in one place, then you may undermine your potential for growth. This fear may keep you in a relationship that you want to leave, for example, or keep you in a dead-end job.

Itching skin can be your body's way of telling you that, spiritually, you are "itching" to move on to the next exciting step in your life. Before you search for treatments and cures, take time to listen to your body and contemplate the message it is trying to give you. Visualization and meditation, described later in this chapter, can be helpful.

Skin Allergy: Your Own Unique Triggers

Like other allergies, the exact causes of skin allergy are a mystery. Certainly, coming in contact with certain foods or chemicals can cause allergic dermatitis. And sunlight can cause hives. However, why some individuals experience these symptoms and others don't remains an unanswered question. Heredity has a role here, especially in eczema. And as discussed earlier, emotions also play a role.

The natural treatments described in this chapter take a range of approaches to skin allergy. Depending on what triggers your own symptoms, some treatments will be more helpful than others. The best way to find out what works for you is to try a few of them out—in the process of discovering what works for you, you may also learn more about your own skin allergy triggers.

NATURAL TREATMENTS FOR SKIN ALLERGIES

Acupressure

Acupressure practitioners view stress and tension as factors causing skin allergies. Stress and tension can be relieved by using the body's pressure points to relax muscular tension. Practitioners also use local points, or pressure points near the affected areas, to help increase circulation. Additional pressure points are used to stimulate the organs and glands related to healthy skin. The practitioner will also use the tonic points, located in the lower back, to stimulate the immune system and the adrenal glands.

Points all over the body can be used for the relief of skin allergies. Here are a few acupressure exercises that you may want to try on your own. See diagrams on pages 384–387.

Eczema One of the acupressure points useful in relieving eczema is the Sea of Vitality (B 23), located in the lower back. To locate these points, reach behind your back at waist level, between the second and third lumbar vertebrae, and count two to four finger widths away from your spine. Use the backs of your hands and rub this area for at least one minute. Breathe deeply and calmly. Rubbing the Sea of Vitality point brings calm and promotes healing and relief of your symptoms.

Another relief for eczema involves using a pressure point below your knee, called the Three Mile point (St 36). This point is located four finger widths below the kneecap toward the outside of the shinbone. Sit upright in a chair and stretch one leg out in front of you. Use your thumb to firmly rub the Three Mile Point on the opposite leg. Use an up-and-down motion. You will know if you've found the right spot if the muscle below this point flexes as you rub. Continue this action for at least one minute, breathing deeply, then repeat it on the other leg.

Conditioning Your Skin   To enhance the overall condition of your skin, use the kidney 2 and 3 points. Pressing these points stimulates the release of the body's internal cortisol. Pressing the LI 4 and LI 11 points releases heat from the body.

Acupuncture

Acupuncture is very effective in treating some skin allergies. Acupuncturists believe that imbalances in lung energy can manifest as skin allergies. In addition, skin allergies may be related to heat from within the body being expressed to the surface, or to various imbalances in the circulatory system.

Affirmations

Skin allergies can have a strong emotional component, with feelings like stress and anger often leading to skin eruptions. When you are reacting to stress by feeling attacked, you send signals to your body, consciously or unconsciously, to get ready for skin allergy symptoms. Affirmations, or self-talk, are messages that we give ourselves that define our expectations in a given situation. And these affirmations can be positive or negative, depending on what you expect. Negative affirmations create an environment for skin allergy symptoms.

You can counteract these negative affirmations with positive ones that define your expectations for an empowered, symptom-free existence. When your allergies are bothering you, you can also use positive self-talk. You can use affirmations that remind you that you do not have to be a victim, redefining an allergen as just a neutral substance that is out there, and that you don't have to react to it. Here are a few affirmations to use for skin allergies:

- I am calm and peaceful. I don't need to scratch and harm myself to feel better.
- My skin is glowing with health. I feel protected.
- I accept my feelings and am not afraid of them.

Create affirmations that work with your specific symptoms and the situations that cause them. Write the affirmations on paper or on small cards, and keep them handy as reminders of positive self-talk. You may even want to tape them up over your kitchen sink or near the bathroom mirror to keep yourself focused.

Aromatherapy

The essential oils of aromatherapy can be useful in treating the symptoms associated with skin allergies and eczema, while also promoting general well-being and a sense of calmness. The scent of some of these oils can be inhaled, allowing them to stimulate the brain cells of the olfactory membrane and sending messages of healing to the central nervous system. It is through inhaling that relaxation and peace of mind are often achieved, and this state of mind can counteract a sense of irritation and the need to scratch, both of which are often associated with skin allergy. Other essential oils can be applied directly to the skin to relieve symptoms, through hot and cold compresses or in lotions and salves. Some essential oils can also be applied directly to the skin or used in bathwater.

The services of an aromatherapist will be particularly helpful in treating skin allergies and eczema, because the practitioner will be able to provide you with mixtures concocted with your specific needs and symptoms in mind. This expertise will be invaluable in the preparation of lotions and salves. While you may have some success from reading an aromatherapy book, the practitioner will add a degree of knowledge and experience that will increase the potential of the essential oils in relieving your symptoms. And relief is the key word with aromatherapy—its application can reduce the effects of your skin allergies. Aromatherapy is also useful in promoting the general health of your skin, adding a vitality that helps strengthen your system so that outbreaks are not as frequent.

Here are some essential oils used in aromatherapy that you can apply at home:

Bergamot   The bergamot tree, grown in Italy and Africa, is a member of the citrus family. The essential oil of the bergamot, which has a fruity aroma, is noted for its calming effect and, when added to an aroma lamp, has been used in treating anxiety and depression. Bergamot is also useful in treating eczema and other skin problems like psoriasis. To treat eczema, you can apply it to your skin. It must, however, be heavily diluted—.5 to 1 percent—in a base oil. Improperly diluted bergamot, when applied to the skin, can cause overpigmentation and may even degenerate into malignant melanomas. If you aren't sure of how to achieve a proper dilution, it is best to work with an aromatherapist.

Chamomile Chamomile is associated with relaxation and the promotion of well-being and is often consumed as a tea. The essential oil of chamomile has these same properties, and it is useful in treating conditions related to nervousness and anxiety, including both stomach and skin disorders. Chamomile can lessen the symptoms of eczema and hives. A few drops can be added to bathwater, it can be used in a massage oil, and a few drops can be applied to the affected areas in a diluted form. Additionally, a few drops can be added to an aroma lamp. Consult an aromatherapist before taking chamomile essential oil internally.

Immortelle Immortelle oil is noted for helping people to look within themselves and achieve awareness. It also has a history of being used as a treatment for disorders of the skin, lymphatic system, and mucous membranes, particularly disorders resulting from irritants in the environment. Immortelle is helpful for treating allergy-related rashes and eczema, often in conjunction with lavender and rockrose. Immortelle can be used in an aroma lamp, in a bath, or diluted in a base oil (with the assistance of an aromatherapist).

Jasmine Jasmine, a member of the olive family, is known to promote self-confidence, deepen moods, and open one up to sensual love. It is also useful in treating ailments related to the emotions, including skin allergies, dermatitis, and eczema. Jasmine oil can be used in an aroma lamp, in a bath, or in a lotion, but should not be used internally. Jasmine oil is also very expensive.

Lemon   The essential oil of lemon can be highly effective in treating skin conditions like eczema in which itching is present. Just add a few drops of lemon oil to a sponge bath, and washing will bring a sense of relief to itchy, irritated skin.

Bath Mixtures to Promote Healthy Skin   Essential oils and some natural ingredients can be used in your bath to help you relax and add vitality to your skin. A few drops of honey in your bathwater nourishes your skin and acts as an antiinflammatory agent. To soften the skin, add four or five tablespoons of sweet cream to your bath, with a few drops of a fragrant oil such as rosemary or orange.

Salt baths have the added benefit of helping to remove toxic substances from your body and strengthening the immune system. Add sea salt to your bath, with a few drops of an essential oil such as lemon, eucalyptus, lime, or lavender to add fragrance.

Always use these mixtures in a peaceful and quiet setting, behind a closed door where you can soak and not be disturbed. And keep an eye on water temperature. Heat the water to a temperature that is comfortable for you— don't force yourself into scalding water.

As with other natural treatments, aromatherapy is not a cure. It can be useful in treating symptoms and promoting healthier skin, but it will not cure your skin allergies. If symptoms persist, or if you have an allergic reaction to one of the essential oils, discontinue its use immediately.

Botanical Medicine

Herbal preparations can have a wonderful effect on skin allergies. In fact, many of the skin preparations available in health food stores contain a substantial amount of herbs. With a couple of good recipes from a botanical medicine book you can begin to create your own herbal skin treatments, and your botanical medicine practitioner can take this treatment a step further by drawing on his or her reservoir of experience to formulate preparations that are unique to your specific makeup and needs.

The botanical medicine approach to skin allergies is focused both on treatment of the symptoms as well as enhancing the natural vitality and resiliency of the skin. A practitioner will view your skin allergies first as a manifestation of the toxins that are running through your system, with hives and dermatitis, for example, being the way in which your specific toxins are showing up on the outside. The treatment approach will therefore begin with herbs that detoxify your system and cleanse your blood, administered both externally and internally. Treatment of your specific symptoms would then be the secondary concern of a botanical medicine approach, based on the assumption that once the toxins are removed, the symptoms of illness will subside. Strengthening your internal organs, especially those that might be associated with your skin ailments, would also be a concern.

Your skin allergies are most likely caused by allergens in your environment. According to the philosophy of selecting your treatment from the same environment that is causing you distress, you should choose from among herbs grown in your region and use them to create tonics for building your system up, as well as using emollients and lotions that will have a soothing and healing action on your skin. Because your skin allergies may return, you should consider always using herbal preparations. Toxins may take years to build up in your system, and the process of returning balance and vitality may also be a relatively long process.

Work with a botanical medicine practitioner in determining the causes of your skin allergies. If the allergies are related to poor circulation, you may need to add warmth to your system through herbs like ginger. Inflammation, however, is a hot condition, and you may need to cool your system down through cooling herbs like dandelion. Your practitioner can make this determination by meeting with you a few times and learning more about your symptoms and when they occur, as well as observing your overall condition. Alterative herbs, which alter conditions like skin irritations, will be especially useful in treating your condition; emollient herbs will soothe and protect your skin, particularly during an allergic reaction; and sedative herbs will have a calming effect on you, which can help reduce the need to scratch. A practitioner might also prescribe other types of herbs, such as laxatives, to help cleanse your body of toxins.

Herbal Treatments and Remedies for Skin Allergies
Your botanical medicine practitioner can devise a treatment plan that is geared specifically toward both the condition of your skin and the symptoms of your skin allergies. In the meantime, here are some of the herbs that are most useful in skin-related treatments and remedies, and methods for trying them on your own at home.

Burdock The herb derived from the roots and seeds of the burdock plant is especially useful in treating skin conditions. In the first place, burdock taken internally is an excellent cleanser of the blood and the lymphatic system, and has been used with much success in clearing up rashes, hives, and eczema. Burdock also contains iron, so it strengthens the blood and, because it detoxifies the liver, it also has a relaxing effect. When using burdock externally to treat skin conditions, it is best applied as an oil. You can either purchase burdock oil from a health food store, or from a practitioner, or follow the directions on page 290 for creating your own supply.

Marshmallow   Marshmallow is derived from the roots of the plant. When used in tea, marshmallow acts as a tonic to strengthen bodily fluids and enhance internal vitality. This can help fortify you against the toxins that can lead to allergic reaction and skin problems. Marshmallow can also be used externally, in a poultice, to treat skin eruptions.

To make a tea with marshmallow or to use marshmallow herb in a poultice, follow the steps on page 291.

Comfrey   Comfrey comes from the root and leaves of the comfrey plant, and is known to promote the growth of cells, while also acting to moisten and lubricate as well as soothe inflamed skin. As such, it is especially good for treating eczema.

To make a salve of comfrey, follow the steps on page 188. Applying the salve directly on the irritated areas should quickly relieve the symptoms. Comfrey can also be used in a poultice, prepared by following the same directions as in creating a marshmallow herb poultice (see page 291).

Licorice   Skin allergies often flare up as a reaction to stress. Licorice can be used to help counteract stress by providing you with a sense of well-being, harmony, and relaxation. Licorice also has a rejuvenating and strengthening effect on the whole body. Licorice herb can be consumed in a tea, made with two to three slices per cup. Drink two or three cups of licorice tea per day.

Working with Your Botanical Medicine Practitioner Your botanical medicine practitioner will want to meet with you and learn as much as possible about how and when your skin allergy symptoms appear, as well as assess the overall condition of your body to gain an understanding of what systems may be out of balance. According to botanical medicine, skin problems are often related to problems of the colon and lungs. Once an assessment is made, your practitioner will develop a treatment routine and instruct you on how to get started. Adjustments will be made in additional sessions, after you have had time to decide if the treatment is helping you or if you are having negative reactions. Make sure you report any problems to your practitioner. If you are also receiving medical treatment for your skin allergies, you may also want to discuss your herbal treatments with your physician to make sure any external preparations will not interact with topical medications you are also using.

Skin allergies can also be the result of the kinds of foods we are eating, and this possibility will most likely be taken into account by your practitioner. Botanical medicine practitioners view the consumption of meat, eggs, and stimulants as creating imbalances that act as triggers for skin allergy. He or she will probably ask you about the kinds of foods you are eating, and may recommend that you include more fruits, vegetables, and whole grains in your diet.

Homeopathy

Homeopathy views all allergies as the result of an imbalance in the system as a whole, which has resulted in oversensitivity. In the case of skin allergies, the oversensitivity may lead to symptoms like hives, contact dermatitis, and eczema. And as with other allergies, the first and foremost homeopathic remedy is basic common sense. Substances that appear to cause allergies should be carefully avoided. This is especially true for contact dermatitis, which can be caused by contact with jewelry, certain plants, chemicals, and other common household substances.

Homeopathic medicine does offer a range of remedies for allergies related to the skin. Diagnosis of these ailments is focused on the appearance of the skin irritation, associated bodily sensations like sensitivity to cold or heat, and also how the symptoms actually occurred in the first place. Based on these factors, homeopathic medicine offers remedies that can be taken internally as well as applied to the skin. Homeopaths discourage the use of hydrocortisone, a commonly used over-the-counter remedy, because they view it as an overly potent drug that is absorbed into the circulation system and can lead to other imbalances. Likewise, the use of calamine lotion is discouraged because it masks symptoms.

Homeopaths first advise their patients to try to figure out what caused the allergic reaction and to avoid it for a week or two, to see if the symptoms clear up on their own. However, the underlying causes of the symptoms can also be treated, especially if they are severe enough to interfere with sleep and other activities. The following are some of the more widely used homeopathic remedies for skin allergies.

Rhus Toxicodendron   Rhus toxicodendron, derived from poison ivy, is useful for treating reactions to poison ivy and sumac, and other types of contact dermatitis. Symptoms that are amenable to treatment by Rhus toxicodendron include burning, itching, and fluid-filled skin eruptions that seem to be worse at night, in open air, and from lying in a warm bed. The rash also worsens after scratching, which may be relieved after immersion in very hot water. Feelings of restlessness and irritability are also clues that Rhus toxicodendron might be a good match with this set of symptoms.

Croton Tiglium   An allergic reaction in which the skin is inflamed and blistered but not itching might call for Croton tiglium. A rash requiring Croton tiglium is also itchy, and it might first be relieved by scratching it a bit. However, this action causes the rash to become so inflamed that even touching it lightly causes pain. Additionally, a rash treatable by Croton tiglium will usually be worse around the eyes, on the scalp, and in the genital area.

Other homeopathic remedies are also useful in treating contact dermatitis, with each prescription based on differences in the appearance and associated symptoms of this ailment. Bryonia, for example, is prescribed for a rash that includes dry bumps accompanied by feelings of irritability. Anacardium is used when symptoms include blisters filled with a yellow fluid.

Apis   Apis is used in treating hives that are extremely itchy and made worse by exposure to warmth, through exercise, for example, or due to a change in the weather. Emotions associated with these hives include sadness and depression, as well as irritability. Also, symptoms often appear first on the right side of the body, and gradually move to the left, and seem to respond positively when exposed to cold temperatures.

While Apis is used most often, Urtica urens, from stinging nettle, and Rhus toxicodendron, from poison ivy, may also be helpful.

No more than three doses of any of these medicines should be taken per day, and they should generally be used for up to three days, or until there is noticeable improvement.

Eczema, which sometimes accompanies respiratory symptoms, is often treated with medicines aimed at curing respiratory ailments. Homeopaths might treat eczema with sabadilla, for example, arsenicum, or Wyethia, depending on the specific range of respiratory symptoms accompanying eczema.

Working with a Homeopathic Physician   Skin allergies are difficult for the layman to treat because the selection of homeopathic medicine is based on subtle differences between groups of related symptoms. For example, it is difficult for a layman to distinguish among various types of blisters or bumps. Thus, it is best to work under the guidance of a qualified homeopathic practitioner.

Meditation

Stress is a major factor, though difficult to measure, in skin allergies. Meditation is widely recognized as an excellent way to relieve stress by creating a sense of inner peace. And when you feel an allergic reaction coming on, or are in the midst of one, creating a sense of peace and relaxation will also calm the immune system. To learn more about meditation, see pages 159–161.

Naturopathy

The guiding principles of naturopathy are described in Chapter 3. Naturopaths view allergies as being rooted in the digestive system and therefore caused at least in part by reactions to food. Skin allergies are no exception, particularly in regard to eczema and hives, the skin allergies that naturopathy most directly addresses.

Naturopaths view eczema as being caused in part by heredity. It may also be related to an immune system weakness, including an impaired ability to fight off bacteria- and virus-related skin diseases. Also, as with other allergies, low stomach acidity can also be a cause. The itching that accompanies eczema may also be caused by stress. The naturopathic approach to treating eczema is based on dealing with these causes.

The causes of hives can be both physical and nonphysical. Physical causes include contact with jewelry, for example, or bedding, as well as coming in contact with heat or cold. Naturopaths view the nonphysical causes of hives as including drugs like penicillin and aspirin that in some individuals cause the formation of antibodies. Consuming food colorings, artificial flavorings, preservatives, and other additives, can also cause hives.

Because eczema and hives are often related to food allergies, a first defense prescribed by the naturopath would be to use the elimination diet to discover the cause of your allergy, and then exclude it from your diet. The elimination diet consists mainly of fish, bananas, rice, potatoes, broccoli, and cabbage. These foods are not likely to result in allergic reactions, and will provide nourishment while the toxins caused by other foods are gradually eliminated from the system. You might stay on this diet for a week or more, at which point additional foods can be introduced, one every day or two. You can look out for any reactions to these foods. If allergic symptoms occur, the new food can be withdrawn. This requires careful record keeping, but it is an excellent way of designing a diet that works for you.

Eczema Nutritional supplements are also used in treating eczema. For example, people with eczema often have a deficiency in essential fatty acids, which results in a decrease in the ability to fight off inflammation, so evening primrose oil might be given to balance this deficiency and relieve symptoms. Eating more fish or using a fish oil supplement might also be recommended for their antiallergy and antiinflammatory effects, as would taking bioflavonoids. Vitamin A helps to enhance the overall healthiness of the skin. Zinc might also be prescribed, in part because it helps to enhance the production of hydrochloric acid in the stomach.

A naturopath might also prescribe botanical medicines to treat your eczema. Vaccinium myrtillus, from blueberry leaf, and Prunus spinosa, from blackthorn, are used to inhibit the production of histamines and serve as antiinflammatories. Burdock root also has a direct healing effect on eczema. Licorice and chamomile can be used in preparations that offer temporary relief.

Naturopaths believe that cortisone has long-term negative effects on the body. Using cortisone on eczema continues the cascade effect that begins with antibiotics. Whereas antibiotics for ailments like ear infections interfere with the digestive system and ultimately result in the histamines being sent to the skin, cortisone sends the histamines on to the lungs, where the result may be allergic rhinitis and asthma.

Naturopaths also recommend the use of a nonoily zinc ointment to relieve the itching associated with eczema, and that only mild soaps be used.

Hives In treating hives, the primary thrust of naturopathic treatment is diet. Naturopaths generally begin with the elimination diet to discover any foods, and food additives, that may be causing these symptoms. Vitamin B_{12} is often prescribed as well, to correct what may be a deficiency in people who suffer from hives. Relaxation, to reduce stress, is also an important component in treating hives, and naturopaths will often recommend relaxation or meditation tapes.

When working with a naturopath, follow the same precautions as with other practitioners. If your condition is at all life threatening, make sure you work closely with your medical doctor to make sure the two approaches to treatment do not conflict. Modifications to your diet, natural herb-based skin remedies, and the practice of meditation, visualization, and other stress-reducing techniques can often add a positive new dimension to your life.

Nutrition

The food you eat can be a definite trigger for skin allergies, especially eczema. Or food may have no effect at all, and the symptoms may be caused by substances like house dust, wool, pollen, and a host of other allergens. However, as with other allergies, eating a diet loaded with chemicals can increase your oversensitivity to allergens so that you are that much more susceptible.

Consulting a nutritionist can get you started in the right direction on learning more about the relationship between what you eat and your skin allergy symptoms. Most likely, you will need to start with an elimination diet to give your system a few days to detoxify. You will lower your overall level of sensitivity by eating foods that should not trigger your allergies. For example, if you suspect that lamb may induce eczema, your elimination diet will not include lamb, though it may be reintroduced at a later time to see how great a role it plays. The same is true with eggs, nuts, or other foods that are known to provoke skin allergies.

These foods can be placed on the forbidden list and then gradually reintroduced, one at a time. If you are being treated for skin allergies by a medical doctor, make sure that he or she is aware of any new diets you are trying.

Psychotherapy

Skin allergy sufferers often report feeling an emotion like anger or fear before breaking out in a rash accompanied by itching, burning, and discomfort. And digging and scratching at your skin eruptions can be a form of self-destructive behavior. Yet avoiding these outbreaks, even when the emotional cause is obvious, is not at all simple.

Psychotherapy is extremely helpful in getting to the root of the emotions that may be causing skin allergy symptoms. With a therapist, you'll talk about the fears you have, bad childhood experiences, the situations in life that are causing you to experience anger or frustration. As you begin to understand your emotions and how to cope with them, you may be able to prevent attacks of hives or eczema.

Psychotherapy, in whatever form you choose, is going to be hard work. Most likely, you'll work one-on-one with a therapist, meeting once or twice a week to talk about your life. You may also want to think about group psychotherapy, especially in a support group with other individuals whose internal conflicts sometimes result in physical symptoms. In any case, make sure you find a therapist with whom you feel comfortable. Be patient as you move forward in psychotherapy, being mindful that you won't uncover the answers overnight.

Reflexology

Reflexology practitioners view skin allergies as the result of internal imbalances caused by the buildup of toxins in your body. Reflexologists treat skin allergy by focusing on the specific imbalances. While imbalances in any number of organs can result in skin problems, those most often involved in skin allergy include the kidneys and lymphatic system. The kidneys can become overloaded with waste and toxic materials, and as a result the blood is not properly cleansed. The lymphatic system can also become impaired, which interferes with its ability to remove toxic wastes from the body. These conditions can contribute to the oversensitivity that leads to allergic reactions.

A visit to a reflexologist would include work on the reflex points that correspond to kidneys and lymphatic systems, as well as other organs to provide a health-giving sense of balance to the whole system. Here are some examples of how a reflexologist might treat your kidneys and lymphatic system. You may want to try these techniques at home with a partner.

The Kidneys   The kidney reflex areas are located on the hands and feet. This area is on the palms of the hands, inside of the tendon to the thumb, just below the index finger. On the feet, the kidney reflex area is in the middle of the arch, almost at the center of the sole.

To apply reflexology to the hand, locate the kidney reflex area and press it with the thumb of the other hand. Press it lightly the first time, release it slightly, press again, this time a bit more firmly. Repeat this action seven times, increasing the pressure each time.

To apply reflexology to the feet, locate the kidney reflex area in the arch of your foot on the sole and press it with the thumb of your other hand. Use the same technique as you did with your hand, pressing lightly, releasing, then pressing more firmly. Do this seven times, gradually increasing the pressure.

Remember that you have two kidneys. Massage both feet and both hands.

The Lymphatic System The reflex points that correspond with the lymphatic system are located on both the hands and feet. On the hands, these points are located on the back, where the hand meets the wrist, and extend like a bracelet from the outer edge of the hand to the inner edge. On the foot, the lymphatic system reflex point is located on top of the foot, at the bend where the feet meet the ankle, from the outside of the ankle around to the inside.

To use the hands, place the index and middle fingers on the reflex area and move along it in a circular motion. Since this reflex area is shaped like a band or bracelet, move along it in small, rolling circles, from one end to the other. Start out gently and when you reach the end of the band, start back at the beginning. Slightly increase the pressure on each pass along the area, for a total of seven repetitions. Don't press too hard.

You can use a very similar technique on your feet. Use your index and middle fingers in a circular motion along the reflex area, starting on the inner ankle bone and moving across the top of the foot to the outer ankle bone. Repeat this action seven times, gradually increasing the pressure each time.

As with other reflexology exercises, it is important to massage the reflex areas on both hands, and then on both feet. Inhale as you press a reflex point, and exhale as you relax the pressure.

Using   Reflexology   for   Your   Skin   Allergies
Reflexology is not useful as an instant relief for the flare-up of a rash. Instead, it should be applied gradually, and at regular intervals as a means of balancing the energy in your system and increasing your ability to relax. Over time, you may begin to see specific results as you gain more control over the frequency and intensity of your symptoms. In any case, reflexology is useful as a calming and relaxing massage.

While you can pick up a book on reflexology and make use of some of the basic techniques, it is best to work with a practitioner, at least at the beginning. The practice of reflexology includes specific positioning of the thumb and fingers, and if you do it improperly you risk not gaining the full benefit. A practitioner can show you a few basic techniques to use at home; you may also want to take a class.

Visualization

There are two things that can make your contact dermatitis, or eczema, or other type of rash even worse. The first is scratching, though with the intense itchiness that these conditions can create, the desire to scratch can become almost uncontrollable, especially when scratching brings so much temporary relief. The other thing that can worsen your skin allergy is stress, with feelings like anger and frustration often causing a new outbreak of symptoms. Visualization can help you create an atmosphere of healing and maintain a relaxed state.

Visualization is based on the philosophy that what you feel on the inside may be reflected on the outside. If you are seething with anger, fear, depression, or any number of negative emotions, skin allergies may be a direct reflection of this state of mind. A patch of eczema can be a reflection of an even larger patch of anger that you are trying to hold back. Visualization is an antidote to the toxic images you are carrying around. It's a means of replacing negative images with images of relaxation and healing— and healthy skin.

When you feel your skin starting to itch, or otherwise feel uncomfortable, find a calm, quiet location. Sit up straight in a comfortable chair, or lie flat on your back on the floor. You may want to play some soft music in the background or use an aroma lamp with a soothing scent.

Visualization begins with relaxation, because you can't focus your mind until you have cleared the chaos out of the way. Meditation techniques can help you relax. Try concentrating on your breathing, counting the inhalation and exhalation. Once your mind is relaxed, you introduce desired images.

Visualize your skin feeling soft and cool, perhaps as someone rubs lotion into it to get rid of the burning and itching. Imagine your skin healing, the bumps and raw spots gradually fading away. Visualize lying on a beach, or in a field, with the sunlight shining on your skin, cooled by a gentle breeze.

When you visualize your skin allergy symptoms, imagine them as ugly blobs that you want to disappear. For example, imagine a big dark stain on a swath of white silk that slowly fades away. Or think of a large patch of mud in the middle of a beautiful bright green lawn, and imagine yourself planting grass seed in the mud and tending the area until the mud is replaced by grass. Imagine your skin allergies as dark, oppressive colors that are replaced by bright, life-giving colors.

Visualize yourself relaxed, surrounded by people who

wish you the best in life. Imagine yourself at one with your surroundings, trusting and being trusted, safe and secure.

Remember that visualization is a preventive measure. Practice it daily to maintain both your sense of calm and the flow of healing.

CHAPTER TEN

Food Allergies

The old cliché, "one man's meat is another man's poison" was never more true than when applied to the problem of food allergies. If you have an allergy to one food or another, and up to five percent of the population does, you've probably watched someone enjoy eating a food that can make you sick simply by looking at it. Like other allergies, food allergies vary widely among individuals, both in terms of the foods that cause reactions and how severe these reactions can become. Food allergies, and what you can do about them, are described in this chapter.

Symptoms of a Food Allergy

A wide range of physical symptoms, from minor to severe, can result from food allergies. However, it's important to keep in mind that these symptoms can also result from viruses and other ailments, as well as from exposure to nonfood allergens. The major food-related allergy symptoms are listed below. Pay close attention not only to the symptoms but also the spans of time in which these symptoms generally appear.

Respiratory Wheezing, runny and itchy or blocked-up nose, bronchitis, and red, runny eyes. Asthma can also be triggered by a food allergy. These symptoms will usually occur within an hour of eating a food to which you are allergic.

Gastrointestinal Colitis, cramps, diarrhea, nausea, ulcers, bed-wetting, gallstones, and vomiting. Symptoms like heartburn and indigestion could occur within half an hour, but may not manifest themselves for another two or three days.

Skin Eczema, sores in the mouth, rashes and hives, persistent itches and soreness. Symptoms like hives and rashes may occur within six to twelve hours.

Muscles and Joints Arthritis, aches and pains with no apparent specific cause. These may occur within forty-eight to ninety-six hours.

Heart and Circulation Racing pulse, spasms and pains that appear similar to angina or heart attack, high blood pressure, flushing or fainting, and migraine. Headache may generally occur within one hour.

Thinking and Emotions Depression, panic attacks, feeling manic, difficulty in concentrating, hyperactivity. The time span for these symptoms will vary, depending in part on your overall mental state.

Have you found that some foods bother you whenever you come in contact with them, while others bother you only at times? Allergic reactions to foods are not always predictable in terms of how quickly the symptoms appear, how severe they are, and when they disappear. For example, you may have to eat a large quantity of a food for it to cause an allergic reaction. Or a food may cause an allergic reaction only when other allergens are present in the air, such as ragweed.

There are actually four types of food allergies, based on the kinds of symptoms experienced during a reaction. These four types are described below.

Fixed Reaction The fixed reaction is the most common type and is almost easy to predict. Just as the term implies, a fixed reaction is one that occurs every time a specific food is eaten. For example, eating a strawberry may directly result in a case of hives. Fixed reactions can happen right after you eat the offending food, even within seconds, but a fixed reaction can also be delayed, even for a day or two, as the allergens travel through your bloodstream.

Cumulative Reaction Cumulative reactions result from a buildup of allergens in your system. For example, eating a food such as strawberries every day over a few days may result in a cumulative reaction, with your body finally storing up enough of the allergens to react. It may take as long as a week or more for your body to ingest enough allergens for a cumulative reaction.

Also, one specific food allergen may not cause a reaction but, when combined with others, the result can be more pronounced. An example of a cumulative reaction might result from sensitivities to both strawberries and cantaloupe. Eating foods that you are allergic to during the spring, when pollen and grass allergens are present in the environment, can also result in a cumulative reaction if you are allergic to all of these substances.

Variable Reaction Food allergies are not always predictable in that a specific food can cause an allergic reaction on some occasions but not on others. Factors such as your state of mind and how stressed out or depressed you might be feeling can affect your reactions to food. The environment, including the presence of pollution, can cause you to be more sensitive to food allergens.

Addiction   Foods can also be addictive, further complicating the treatment process because you may swing back and forth between extreme craving followed by physical reactions that subside only to be replaced by more craving. Overeating foods like sugar, salt, or wheat can be a form of addiction when these foods result in allergy symptoms or other illnesses.

As you explore natural treatments for your food allergy, you will want to keep in mind the kinds of symptoms that occur, as well as what seems to lead up to a food reaction. You may treat some food allergies by simply avoiding certain foods. For example, when you're out with friends, you may want to avoid the strawberry shortcake and order a different dessert.

Unfortunately, treating many food allergies is not that simple, particularly if the food allergy is cumulative in nature, and therefore less predictable. Natural medicine alternatives that strengthen your body and build up your gastrointestinal system, such as botanical medicine and homeopathy, will be helpful here. Relaxation techniques like visualization, and emotional supports like psychotherapy and twelve-step groups, can also help.

In any case, take some time to understand your food allergies as much as possible as you consider alternate treatment methods. And follow a few commonsense guidelines, described later in this chapter.

Another Immune System Overreaction

Food allergies are similar to other allergies in that they are most likely caused by an immune system overreaction. The body produces antibodies, particularly IgE, in unhealthy quantities when the wrong food is introduced to the system. As with other allergies, histamine is produced. The blood vessels widen, and smooth muscles contract so that affected skin areas become red, itchy, and swollen. IgE antibodies in the tissues and secretions result in the classic food allergy symptoms like hives, diarrhea, and swollen membranes.

But why does the immune system in some people—and maybe you're one of those people—overreact to certain foods? Food allergies are in many ways as much a mystery as allergic rhinitis and skin allergies. However, certain factors like heredity may be a factor. For example, if one or both of your parents have an allergy, chances are high that you will have the same allergy. Excessive exposure to a certain food can also result in allergy. Some Japanese, for example, are allergic to rice, while fish allergy is common among Scandinavian people.

Your reactions to a certain food can also be affected by your overall physical condition at the time. If you have an upset stomach or are experiencing other allergy symptoms like hay fever, you may also be more susceptible to food allergy.

Another important factor in food allergy is emotion. Your overall state of mind—if you feeling angry, for example, or stressed out—can also cause you to overreact.

When you are feeling angry or otherwise upset, do you feel a clutching in your stomach and a loss of appetite? On the other hand, are you a depression eater, looking to food as a means of providing yourself with some needed comfort? The connection between appetite and eating is complicated, yet undeniable. If you suffer from food allergy, the role of emotion in your symptoms is even more complicated. When stress is mixed with a food that tends to cause allergy symptoms, even more pronounced symptoms can result because your defenses are already compromised as a result of the stress. Natural medicine offers a range of options to soothe the emotions that can be a prelude to an allergic reaction.

Not All Reactions Are Allergies

It's important to keep in mind that not all reactions to food are a result of a food allergy. Food can affect you in a variety of ways. You may find that you have an aversion to a certain food for psychological reasons. And while you may not be sure of these reasons, you just know that when you see or smell this food, you have an urge to run in the other direction, or even to become ill. Or certain foods or spices may cause a burning stomach.

Your body can also have an inability to digest certain foods, such as milk, because of an enzyme deficiency. Diabetes or hypoglycemia (low blood sugar) can also interfere with your body's ability to tolerate certain foods. These are food-related problems, but they are not food allergies.

The Major Culprits

Foods that are most likely to cause allergic reactions include:

Milk products   Milk allergies can be found in both children and adults, in addition to an inability to digest lactose.

Wheat Wheat allergy can also result from an intolerance to gluten, which is a part of wheat.

Eggs The white is the part of the egg that most often causes allergies, and may or may not extend to chicken as well.

Nuts Allergic reactions can be caused by certain types of nuts, such as almonds or walnuts.

Vegetables Peas, beans, and tomatoes are the vegetables most likely to cause an allergic reaction, and these reactions can be caused both by inhalation, as when a vegetable is being peeled, as well as by eating.

Meat The meats most likely to cause allergic reactions include beef, pork, and chicken.

Fish and Shellfish Reactions to fish and shellfish can be violent.

Alcohol Allergic reactions to alcoholic beverages are often the result of allergies not only to the alcohol but also to ingredients such as yeast, molasses, sulfites, and malt.

Corn Corn appears in a wide range of foods, including baked goods, corn syrup, sauces, soups, cornstarch, corn oil, so allergic reactions to corn can often crop up unexpectedly.

Caffeine Chocolate, tea, coffee, and soft drinks containing caffeine can cause allergic reactions.

Fruits Citrus fruits as well as apples may cause allergic reactions.

o   o   o

And while foods can result in allergic reactions, the additives in them present yet a whole new set of potential allergens.

Prevention First: Avoid Additives in Food

Some of the main culprits in food allergies are the preservatives and additives found in so many foods. A simple loaf of bread can contain refined wheat flour, a range of preservatives, salt with added iodine, synthetic vitamins, benzoyl peroxide bleach, and other artificial chemicals to keep the dough smooth. And a slice of bread may play a relatively small part in your daily diet. Think of all other packaged and processed foods you consume between breakfast and bedtime.

The following is a list of some of the additives most often used in food and the foods in which they are commonly found.

Aspartame, which is usually referred to by its brand name, NutraSweet, is a low-calorie sweetener used to replace sugar in desserts, sodas, chewing gum, breath mints, candy, and other foods. Aspartame can cause headaches, hives, and swelling of the lips, hands, and eyelids, though these reactions are considered rare.

BHA/BHT are agents that prevent oxygen absorption, referred to as antioxidants. These agents are used in candies, crackers, cereals, and other grain products as a preservative. They can cause headaches and rashes in individuals who are allergic to them and hyperkinesis in children.

Dyes and Coloring are used in foods ranging from bread, ice cream, jam, smoked fish, breakfast cereals, to maraschino cherries. They can cause hives, as well as bronchial congestion.

MSG, or monosodium glutamate, is often found in Chinese, Japanese, and other Asian foods. MSG reactions include headache, diarrhea, sweating, nausea, chest tightness, and a burning sensation along the back of the neck. It is important to note that MSG is used as a flavor enhancer in a wide range of foods, including snack foods and some canned soups and sauces, and not only in Asian foods.

Nitrates/Nitrites are used to preserve, enhance flavor, and provide color to prepared foods. These agents are most commonly found in meat products like hot dogs, ham, preserved meats, as well as in soup mixes. Nitrates and nitrites can cause headaches, nausea, vomiting, hives, cyanosis, and blood pressure disorders.

Parabens, like methyl and sodium benzoate, are used as preservatives. Parabens can cause the skin to swell, burn or itch, and turn red.

Sulfites, like sulfur dioxide and sodium bisulfite, are used both to preserve food as well as sanitize containers for fermented beverages. Sulfites are found in a variety of canned, frozen, and dehydrated food, including dried fruit, processed grain food like crackers and chips, in canned seafood, and in fruit juices, cider, and wine and beer. Sulfites can cause chest tightness, diarrhea, abdominal cramps, rashes, light-headedness, weakness, and an elevated pulse rate.

o   o   o

Clearly, you can't stop eating. You may not even be able to stop eating prepared food. However, if you are experiencing some of the symptoms described above, look closely at the labels of the foods you are eating. And when you start to see a pattern, such as reactions to foods containing sulfites, you can start to treat yourself through avoidance. Read the labels on prepared food before you drop it in your grocery cart. Replace these foods, wherever possible, with natural, organically grown foods, as well as with foods that you have prepared at home.

Guidelines for Defensive Eating

While food allergies are unpredictable in terms of the kinds of foods that cause allergic reactions, the types of symptoms, and when reactions occur, there are still some generally accepted guidelines for helping to keep your food allergies to a minimum. These guidelines are outlined below.

1. Stay away from canned and frozen vegetables. The linings of metal cans, as well as the plastic bags used for storing frozen vegetables, can cause allergic reactions. It is not always possible, or affordable, to purchase only organically grown foods. Still, fresh vegetables are preferable to canned and frozen vegetables.

2. Buy meat from a butcher shop. Meat is often packed in Styrofoam (polystyrene) and polyurethane. These substances are derived from petrochemicals. As much as possible, avoid them by purchasing meat from a butcher shop, where it is wrapped in paper.

3. Avoid processed foods. TV dinners, lunch meat, and other processed foods often contain chemicals,

as well as large amounts of sugar and salt. Avoid these quick solutions and focus on healthy, easy-to-prepare alternatives.

4. Buy spring water. Tap water often contains chlorine as well as pesticides and other chemicals that may have seeped into the water supply. Spring water is available in convenient containers, at a low cost, in most grocery stores.

5. Watch out in restaurants. You can't always be sure of what kinds of preservatives or other additives are contained in food that you haven't purchased for yourself. Be especially careful of salad bars, where the fruits and vegetables may sit for days at a time, and be dipped in chemicals to make them appear fresh.

6. Eat a varied diet. Get a comprehensive list of the basic food groups and, each day, choose different foods from each group. You may discover that you have adopted a pattern of eating foods you are allergic to, a pattern that isn't apparent until you break it with variety.

Discovering Your Food Allergies

Nobody knows as much as you do about your food allergies, yet you may be unsure which specific foods affect you. Before you begin making decisions about treatment alternatives for your food allergies, it is important to learn as much as possible about what you are allergic to and how these allergies affect you. To do your own detective work, the best place to start is a diary.

Grab some paper and make lists of everything you put into your mouth, from the moment you wake up until you go to bed. Remember, everything that passes your lips should be on this list, and make a note of the exact time of day next to each item. Also, keep track of any symptoms you may have. Headaches. Rashes. Nausea. Any of these symptoms should be noted, with the exact time of day that they occur, as well. Remember, as you read earlier in the chapter, various symptoms may take time to show up.

Keep this diary for a couple of weeks and watch for patterns that emerge. Do fruits seem to be associated with hives? Are you getting headaches after eating packaged foods? Also, based on your diary, start exploring the following questions:

Where are you eating your meals? At home? In the car?

Do your eating habits change on weekends? What about brunch?

How much are you snacking? And what are you snacking on?

When are you drinking coffee? Soda? Tea?

What are your eating habits at work? Where are you eating? Outside? In a restaurant? At your desk? Are you eating in a quiet place?

When are you drinking alcohol? At lunch? In the afternoon? Evening? Are you drinking cocktails? Beer? Wine?

Do you eat take-out food at night? TV dinners?

What about dessert?

Do you have a late-night snack? What?

Do some foods taste too rich for you? Do you eat them anyway?

Are you taking vitamins? What kinds?

What about laxatives, decongestants, aspirin, antacids, breath mints, and gum?

Answer these questions carefully, and think about every day of the week. Again, the goal is to look for patterns that might be a key to any allergic reactions you are experiencing. Don't forget that some foods can interact with each other. And alcohol and medicine can complicate the picture.

To help you in this exercise, you might also want to pick up a book that lists foods and provides detailed information on preservatives, potential allergic reactions, and other information such as calorie count.

By understanding what foods you are allergic to, and the kinds of symptoms you have, you are in a better position to begin making decisions about your treatment alternatives.

NATURAL MEDICINE AND FOOD ALLERGY

Natural medicine treats the cause as well as the symptoms of food allergy. A nutritionist, for example, can help you to eliminate allergy-causing foods from your diet and design a diet that better meets your needs. A macrobiotic diet may be one of your options. Naturopathy and homeopathy can provide you with remedies for food-allergy symptoms like gastrointestinal distress. Reflexology and visualization can help you to achieve relaxation and reduce the stress that often makes you more susceptible to food allergy.

The specific foods, or combinations of foods, that cause allergic reactions, the situations in which these reactions occur, and the actual symptoms are different for each food-allergy sufferer. As you read about natural medicine alternatives for your food allergy, keep in mind your own specific situation and the kind of relief you are seeking. Some alternatives will be more helpful than others. And if you are under the care of a medical doctor, communicate with him or her to make sure that any decisions you make do not interfere with other treatment you are receiving.

Acupressure

Acupressure can offer relief for the symptoms of food allergies, including diarrhea and nausea. Treatment includes balancing the digestive system. As such, acupressure can be a good approach to use in conjunction with treatments that deal more directly with food allergies, such as herbalism, nutrition, and botanical medicine. Acupressure is described in more depth in Chapter 3.

Here are some examples of acupressure treatments that you can try on your own:

Diarrhea   Acupressure points useful in relieving diarrhea include St 36, Sp 6 and 9, and CV 6. See diagrams on pages 384–387. Sit up straight in a chair. Reach behind your back at waist level, between the second and third lumbar vertebrae, and count two to four finger widths away from your spine. Use the backs of your hands and rub this area for at least one minute. Breathe deeply and calmly. This action will relax you and promote healing and relief of your symptoms.

Here's another way of doing this exercise. Lie on your back, with your legs bent and your feet flat on the floor. Slowly raise your pelvis, and place your fists underneath your lower back. Position your knuckles between your spine and the muscles of your lower back. Relax down into the fists. Close your eyes and breathe deeply into your stomach.

Digestion Digestion is enhanced through the Three Mile point (St 36), located below your knee. This point is located four finger widths below the kneecap toward the outside of the shinbone. Sit upright in a chair, and stretch one leg out in front of you. Use your index finger to firmly rub the Three Mile point (St 36). Use an up-and-down motion. You will know you've found the right spot if the muscle below this point flexes as you rub. Continue this action for at least one minute, breathing deeply, then repeat it on the other leg.

Abdominal Spasms Abdominal spasms can be relieved through the Center of Power point (CV 12), an acupressure point near your stomach. Lie on your stomach, and slide your right hand underneath your stomach until you locate the point between the bottom of your breastbone and your naval. Then position the palm of your left hand between your pubic bone and belly button (over point CV 4–6). Turn your head to one side. Close your eyes and breathe deeply and slowly. The exercise should have an immediate effect, causing your symptoms to subside within minutes.

Acupuncture

The acupuncture approach to food allergies is to determine, and then resolve, the underlying energetic imbalances that predispose someone to food allergies. These imbalances differ among individuals. A qualified acupuncture practitioner can make this diagnosis and begin a series of treatments.

Affirmations

The use of affirmations, described in Chapter 3, is a way of sending positive healing messages and relaxation directly to your body, especially the areas that are most affected by food allergy.

Here are a few affirmations to use for food allergies:

- I am giving myself permission to enjoy my food.
- I am relaxed and confident, and I am ready to take charge of my life.
- I can easily digest my food. I trust life and release all of my fears.
- I am opening myself up to peace, comfort, and the joy of living.

Create affirmations that counteract the effects of the foods that you seem to be most allergic to or that most directly address your food allergy symptoms, such as hives or diarrhea. Write the affirmations on paper or on small cards, and keep them handy as reminders of positive self-talk. You may also want to record your affirmations on tape and then play it when you're driving or working around the house. The best time to say affirmations is during the morning, when your mind is fresh, as well as in the evening before bedtime.

Aromatherapy

Aromatherapy, described in Chapter 3, can be useful in treating the symptoms associated with food allergies, though it is not a cure for food allergies and may not necessarily be helpful in preventing symptoms. Still, the essential oils used in aromatherapy can be beneficial in alleviating stomach and abdominal cramps. If your food allergies result in rashes, you may also want to refer to Chapter 9 for guidance in using aromatherapy for lessening skin-related symptoms. And because aromatherapy promotes relaxation and feelings of calm and well-being, you can apply it to help yourself reduce the stress that often contributes to a worsening of symptoms.

In treating food allergy symptoms, you can use the essential oils in an aroma lamp, in a bath, or in hot compresses. As stated previously, it is never a good idea to ingest aromatherapy oils without the guidance of an aromatherapist as well as the permission of your physician. Your system may be especially sensitive to the potential toxic effects of the oils.

Here are a few essential oils that are useful in treating gastrointestinal symptoms:

Angelica   The oil of the angelica plant, grown in Eastern Europe, is useful in building physical and mental stamina. When a few drops are used in an aroma lamp, you can receive both the strengthening effects of angelica and relief for nausea. When used internally, angelica stimulates the digestive system and promotes digestion. However, you should use it internally only under the guidance of a qualified practitioner.

Chamomile   One of the major uses of chamomile oil is in relieving the symptoms of stomach and intestinal problems. Place a few drops in an aroma lamp or in a warm bath, and breathe in its calming and healing fragrance. You can also obtain relief from extreme cramps by soaking a compress in hot water with a few drops of chamomile added to it. Make sure the water is comfortably but not excessively hot, and when it cools, soak the compress again in the hot water and reapply it.

Mint   Mint oil is useful in relieving symptoms such as cramps, nausea, and vomiting. Use a few drops of mint oil in an aroma lamp. Mint oil can also be taken internally, though it is important that it be well diluted with water. Again, seek the advice of a practitioner before using it internally.

Botanical Medicine

Botanical medicine can be widely applied in treating food allergies. Herbs can be used to rejuvenate the digestive system, enhancing your ability to withstand the assault on your system that can result from exposure to a food that, for you, acts as an allergen. Herbs can also be used to treat the symptoms of food allergy, from nausea to diarrhea. Additionally, herbs can be used to promote relaxation, helping you to be less sensitive to the food you eat and thus less likely to react. Many of the herbs used in treating food allergies, however, are ingested or administered as enemas or laxatives. Thus, special cautions should be kept in mind. These will be discussed later in this section, but first the benefits.

According to the theory behind botanical medicine, we react to food because of the toxins that have built up in our systems. Chemicals and other food additives, as well as the toxins we are exposed to in the air we breathe, have created a hostile internal environment that is constantly in a reactive mode. Thus, a seemingly innocuous food can set off a violent reaction. And we often continue to add to these toxins by consuming excessive amounts of meat, re-fined sugar, alcohol, and foods treated with pesticides and preservatives. This can lead to a cycle of adverse reactions that we label food allergy.

The herbal treatment for the symptoms of food allergy is the standard three-level approach, as described in

Chapter 3. Herbs would first be administered to promote the elimination of the toxins in the digestive system. This step might include herbs that promote sweating, such as cayenne and peppermint; emetics to induce vomiting, like ipecac; and laxatives such as rhubarb root and senna. Blood purifiers would also be administered. Herbal treatment for the symptoms associated with food allergy might include carminatives such as anise and fennel to relieve gas, and antacids, like slippery elm, to reduce stomach acid. Herbs are also useful in strengthening and energizing your digestive organs so that your symptoms are not as severe and dissipate more quickly.

The following are some of the more commonly used herbs in treating digestive problems, including the symptoms of food allergies, with suggestions on how you can use them at home. Most of these herbs are relatively easy to find.

Anise Aniseed is a warm herb, useful in treating the stomach, liver, and kidneys. You probably have a supply of anise on your spice rack, and are familiar with its spicy taste. Anise warms the digestive system, particularly the abdominal area, and relieves nausea and gas, reduces abdominal pains, and stimulates digestion. The easiest way to administer anise is in a hot cup of tea, using the directions on page 292.

Cayenne Cayenne is a hot herb, known for its stimulating effect on digestion. It can be used in treating cramps and diarrhea, as an appetite stimulant, and for help in dispelling gas. In small doses it is also useful for helping to clear up stomach ulcers. To learn how to administer cayenne, refer to pages 292–293.

Peppermint Peppermint is a useful herb in treating indigestion, helping to relieve gas, vomiting, and nausea. It has a pleasing flavor, and is most often used in a tea. You can make a peppermint tea by using the same method as used in making the anise tea described on page 292. Peppermint tea can also be purchased from a health food store, in loose leaf form or in tea bags. Drink a few cups of peppermint tea, and experience its soothing effect on your digestive system.

Chamomile Chamomile is useful in soothing nervous tension as well as calming the digestive system. It relieves cramps, upset stomach, and gas, and enhances the digestion process. Chamomile also has the added benefit of providing your system with additional calcium.

To make a chamomile tea, follow the instructions for anise tea described on page 292. You can also purchase chamomile tea in a health food or grocery store.

Ginger Ginger has both healing and detoxifying effects on the digestive system, and because it produces a warming energy it can also be used in treating upset stomach and difficulty in digestion. Make a tea with either a few slices of fresh ginger, if available, or an ounce of dried gingerroot, in a pint of water. Drink a cup every two hours or so, until your symptoms disappear.

If your food allergies cause abdominal pain, you can relieve the pain with a ginger compress by following these directions:

1. Make a strong ginger tea.
2. Soak a washcloth in the tea for ten minutes.
3. Remove the washcloth with tongs, wring it out well, and lay it over your abdomen.

4. Cover the washcloth with a dry towel and place a hot water bottle on top of the towel.

5. Leave the compress in place for a half hour.

The ginger compress will have a warming, and therefore soothing, effect on your cramps. Repeat this treatment until your symptoms disappear.

Botanical Medicine and Addiction

Recovering from addiction is a complex process, involving physical, social, psychological, and spiritual factors. There are no quick cures. And botanical remedies do not in general address the issue of alcoholism and other addictions. However, the properties of herbs can be helpful in treating this condition in conjunction with your traditional therapy program. While addiction may not be a result of toxins in the blood, substances like alcohol certainly add toxins, and also impair the functioning of the kidneys, liver, and other organs. Herbs can be used to help remove the toxins from the blood as well as rejuvenate and strengthen these organs. Alcohol also affects the circulatory, digestive, and nervous systems; herbal remedies can help to repair these systems and restore lost energy. Herbs that have a calming and relaxing effect may help to reduce the need to use tranquilizing substances by eliminating the agitated state of mind that often leads to addictive behavior. Also, the herb skullcap has a history of use in treating alcoholism and other addictions.

Botanical medicine used in treating addiction can be beneficial for its restorative properties alone. The following are some of the herbs that you might find helpful in treating addiction and related symptoms, and how you can use them at home. You should check with your treating physician before taking any new remedy.

Skullcap Skullcap is classified as a nervine herb, meaning that it promotes relaxation and reduces nervous tension. Skullcap contains potassium, magnesium, and calcium, and acts directly on the central nervous system to produce its calming effects. Skullcap is useful during withdrawal from substance abuse not only because of its relaxing effects but because it has a detoxification property that helps to lessen the symptoms of withdrawal such as shakiness.

You can take skullcap in a tea made with one teaspoon of tincture of skullcap per cup of hot water, or one ounce of the dry herb per pint of water. If using dry herbs, follow these directions for making herbal tea:

1. Place the skullcap in a teapot.
2. Boil a pint of water in a separate container. When the water starts to boil, pour it over the herb in the teapot.
3. Cover the pot and let the herb steep for fifteen minutes.
4. Strain the herb fragments through cheesecloth or a sieve.

During withdrawal, drink a cup of tea every hour or so. You may be able to purchase a tincture of skullcap from a health food store or from a practitioner. If you are using the tincture during withdrawal, take fifteen drops every couple of hours.

For general use, up to three cups of skullcap tea per day is enough to experience its calming effects.

Withdrawal from the abuse of alcohol is a serious situation and should not be undertaken without being in the care of a physician, if not in a supervised environment. Herbal preparations can help reduce symptoms, but do not replace the need for medical attention.

Burdock The herb from the root and seeds of the burdock plant cleanses the blood, and because it contains iron and other minerals, it also has a strengthening effect on the blood. Burdock is also useful in cleansing the liver and, because it has a diuretic property, also stimulates the flushing of harmful substances from the kidneys. Burdock can be taken in a tea, prepared as follows:

1. Place one ounce of burdock in a pot containing one pint of water.
2. Bring this container of water to a boil, then lower the heat and allow it simmer for approximately one hour.
3. Strain the herb fragments through cheesecloth or use a strainer.

Drink the burdock tea three times per day to experience the detoxifying and rejuvenating effects.

Applying Botanical Medicine to Addiction As described above, botanical medicine treatments for addiction are limited to providing potential relief of withdrawal symptoms, inducing relaxation and peace of mind, and detoxifying and strengthening the system. The restorative effects of herbs can be invaluable, and you can apply herbal remedies on your own to experience these effects. A botanical medicine practitioner can help you to use herbs in combination to optimize the benefits of this approach.

Still, it's important to keep in mind that while an addiction such as alcoholism may have a physical cause, and may indeed be an allergy, treating addiction is a complex process. Herbal preparations cannot take the place of emotional supports like twelve-step groups and therapy. And if you are experiencing withdrawal symptoms, treatment by a physician is also important.

Working with a Botanical Medicine Practitioner

A botanical medicine practitioner will not encourage you to simply treat your food allergy symptoms; instead he or she will talk with you about changes in your diet. You'll be asked a lot of questions about the kinds of foods you're eating before and after you experience allergy symptoms. You may be asked to keep a journal for a few weeks to record every piece of food that you put into your mouth. This information will be used as the basis not only for herbal remedies but also a diet plan.

According to botanical medicine practitioners, foods act the same way as herbs once they are introduced into our systems. Some foods, like meats, have warm or hot energy. Others, like fruit, are neutral or cooling in their effect on the body. If you are eating too much meat, you may be causing your body to react with symptoms associated with food allergy, like abdominal pain and gas. Foods can also be adding toxins to your body. Thus, your symptoms may be not so much the result of a specific food as of overindulgence in certain types of foods. By eating a balanced diet, you also take in a balance of warm and cool energies.

Over time, your botanical medicine practitioner will guide you toward adopting a diet that includes foods from the basic food groups, rich in fruits and vegetables, grains, and nuts, with some dairy and meat products, depending on your lifestyle. He or she may first take measures to counter any current imbalances in your system. For example, you may be instructed to remove meat from your diet for a while, until the body has a chance to rid itself of toxins as well as cool down from the warm energy produced by meat. You may also be instructed to use certain herbal preparations such as ginger with your food to aid in digestion.

Use Caution with Herbs Because many of the herbal remedies for food allergies are taken internally, exercise caution as you use them. Some herbs can have toxic side effects, especially if taken in large doses, and it is advisable to keep internal use to a minimum, outside of standard herbal teas, unless you are consulting a practitioner. Keep in mind that your digestive system is already sensitive, and herbal preparations, if not used carefully, can create additional strain. Also be careful about using laxative herbs as they too can be harsh for your system.

Keep your physician "in the loop" if you choose to become involved in an extensive botanical medicine regimen to ensure that it will not interfere with other medications you are already taking. Also, watch your own reactions carefully. If you find the preparations are making you sick, or if you are having allergic reactions more often, report this to your botanical medicine practitioner so that changes can be made. If symptoms are abnormal and/or severe, also talk to your physician.

Homeopathy

Food allergy, according to homeopathy, results from toxins that have accumulated in the digestive system and created an imbalance. Treatment is aimed at matching symptoms such as vomiting, nausea, and diarrhea with a homeopathic medicine that mimics these symptoms, and helps the body to bring itself back into balance. Additionally, homeopathic remedies can be helpful in creating an environment for healing to take place. The philosophy of homeopathy is described in Chapters 2 and 3.

Homeopathic remedies are often a reliable alternative to chemical-based medications that not only add toxins to the system but mask symptoms that will return once the drug wears off, and which may interfere with natural digestive and healing processes. Many over-the-counter remedies also contain chemicals that can further contribute to the imbalances in your system, which can lead to additional problems.

As with other allergies, a homeopathic physician will sometimes recommend letting food allergy symptoms take their course without any specific intervention. For example, stay away from specific foods that cause allergic reactions, drink plenty of water to replace the loss of fluids that results from diarrhea, and stay warm and comfortable until the symptoms have disappeared. In many situations, this might be all that is necessary.

If the vomiting is more severe, the lining of the stomach is most likely inflamed, perhaps as a result of the allergy. Food and liquid can irritate it further. First, consume a minimal amount of liquids for up to twelve hours, to allow the symptoms to calm down. Then begin to replace the fluids with tiny amounts of clear liquids, such as vegetable broth, juice, or flat soda. Avoid milk and animal products. Over the next day or two, gradually increase the liquids and start to eat solid foods like toast and yogurt.

Food allergies can also result in abdominal pain. This can be treated by resting, and eating small meals of mild food and drinking clear liquids. This will let the symptoms work themselves out. Abdominal pain can also be related to appendicitis rather than a food allergy, and when these pains occur without other symptoms and either continue or worsen, immediate medical attention may be necessary.

Symptoms like abdominal pain, vomiting, and diarrhea

can also be treated with homeopathic medicines. Some of the most commonly used medicines are as follows:

Arsenicum Album Arsenicum is one of the more commonly used homeopathic medicines for treating ailments of the gastrointestinal system with symptoms that include vomiting, diarrhea, and stomach or intestinal pain. Other symptoms that point to the need for arsenicum include fearfulness, exhaustion, and restlessness, as well as extreme thirst and chilliness. These symptoms are worse at night, and eating and drinking quickly result in vomiting. There is burning and cramping in the stomach or abdomen. A fever may be present, but also a feeling of being cold.

Ipecac Ipecac is a useful homeopathic medicine if the major symptom is nausea, with or without diarrhea or vomiting. Ipecac is used by individuals who are most likely not as seriously ill as those needing arsenicum. Nausea continues, even after vomiting, and it is made worse by contact with even the smell of food. Some diarrhea and gas may accompany the nausea.

Colocynthis Colocynthis, derived from bitter cucumber, is indicated if the major symptom is abdominal cramps made worse by eating or drinking. This type of cramps can be relieved through gentle pressure on the abdomen, and warmth. Vomiting may occur if the pain becomes severe enough. Feelings of irritability may also be present.

Belladonna, from deadly nightshade, may also be useful in the early stages of gastrointestinal distress, if the symptoms have come on suddenly.

◦ ◦ ◦

Generally, these medicines should be given once per hour in acute cases until the symptoms begin to subside. Medicines should be given every twelve hours if symptoms are less severe. When using a homeopathic medicine for possible food allergy symptoms, you should notice improvements rather quickly. If not, switch to another homeopathic medicine. Always consult your doctor before taking any new remedies. And again, if symptoms become severe, get medical assistance.

Meditation

As discussed earlier, food allergy symptoms can be made worse by stress and, on the other hand, relieved by relaxation. Meditation helps you to relieve stress by creating a sense of inner peace and relaxation.

The best approach to meditation is to learn a technique and then practice it on a daily basis, even if it is for only a few minutes every day, generally in the morning. The result of this practice is a sense of calm that will stay with you during the remainder of the day. Additionally, with practice you will be able to use your meditation technique to help achieve calm when you suddenly find yourself in a stressful situation, especially one in which you might be more susceptible to food-related allergens. An example of a meditation technique is described in Chapter 4.

Naturopathy

Naturopaths view food allergy as the result of a wide range of causes. Heredity is a factor. The immune system is also a factor, with some foods stimulating the production of histamines which, in turn, can lead to food allergy symptoms. The permeability of the gut is also a factor in food allergy, allowing partially digested protein to cross the intestinal barrier and be absorbed into the bloodstream, leading to the allergy response. Low stomach acidity, another factor, will also result in undigested food entering the bloodstream.

Naturopaths treat food allergy primarily through elimination diets. This begins with a regimen that might consist of lamb, potatoes, bananas, rice, and vegetables such as broccoli and cabbage. These foods are not likely to result in allergic reactions, and will provide nourishment while the toxins caused by other foods are gradually eliminated from the system. Generally, you would stay on this kind of diet for a week or more, at which point additional foods can be introduced, one every day or two. If other allergic symptoms occur, the new food can be withdrawn. This requires careful record keeping, but it is an excellent way of designing a diet that works for you. The elimination diet does work especially well with specific food allergies because the time between when a food first enters the system and subsequently leads to an allergic reaction may be relatively short. As a result, discovering your food allergies may be a relatively simple process.

Naturopaths also recommend the rotary diversified diet for food allergies. This diet helps to keep your food allergy symptoms to a minimum by lessening exposure to the known allergies as well as preventing new ones. Naturopaths believe that if tolerated foods are eaten on a regular basis, new allergies will not be induced. In the rotary diversified diet, the foods that are tolerated are eaten at specific intervals, every four to seven days. With this routine firmly established, foods that have been known to cause allergic symptoms can gradually be introduced. This way, you can begin to again enjoy foods that were previously forbidden.

Because of the possibility of reactions caused by eating foods from the same group, this diet requires some rotation of food groups. This can become a bit complicated until you develop a pattern. Naturopaths who do not specialize in nutrition may bring in another practitioner to help in developing a diet.

Food allergy is often associated with immune system dysfunction. Naturopaths often prescribe nutritional supplements that strengthen the immune system, including selenium, zinc, and B complex.

As with other allergies, the naturopathic treatment for food allergy is holistic. Diet recommendations will be supplemented by stress-reduction techniques, including meditation, as well as supportive counseling, exercise, and possibly some kind of bodywork, with the goal of relieving both your symptoms and helping you to develop a more positive attitude and lifestyle. If you are under the care of a medical doctor, talk to him or her before you make any major changes in your diet. You may already have been tested for allergic reactions to some of the foods you might be eliminating or introducing on the naturopath's recommended diet. Also, if you suffer from diabetes or low blood sugar, make sure you talk to your doctor about any changes to your diet.

Nutrition

Virtually any food you consume can cause an allergic reaction, though some foods, like nuts, citrus fruit, shellfish, and dairy products, are more likely to be allergy triggers. Many natural approaches to treating food allergy are based on relieving symptoms such as nausea, diarrhea, and vomiting. The field of nutrition has a deceptively simple answer to the problem of food allergy—it goes straight to the cause, and then treats the problem through avoidance.

If you are aware of what foods you are allergic to, a nutritionist can help you set up a diet that avoids those specific foods, as well as members of the same food family that may also trigger reactions. If you are unsure of what foods are bothering you, your nutritionist may also develop an elimination diet for you to help you discover your food allergies, and that fits in with your lifestyle and food preferences. Find a nutritionist with experience in treating food allergies and be willing to work closely with him or her, even though that will mean measuring and recording the foods you eat, and also keeping detailed records of any symptoms you experience. While you may learn that you have to avoid some foods that you really enjoy, like ice cream, the freedom from allergy symptoms should more than compensate for the loss.

Having an allergy to some foods, like shellfish, can be life threatening. Not only is absolute avoidance critical but so is the availability of medical attention. Make sure your medical doctor is aware of your food allergies and that medication is available if needed, and communicate with your physician and nutritionist to make sure your treatment is not going in two different directions.

Psychotherapy

Are your food allergies psychosomatic? Has unresolved anger caused you to become allergic, for example, to wheat? Probably not. However, there is a strong connection between your emotions and how you feel about food. Stress, anger, depression . . . they all affect how and what you eat. Addiction can also be a factor in your eating patterns. You can probably remember back to family meals in your childhood, when you felt good about eating, or when you felt too upset to finish your meal. And you can probably remember becoming sick after eating certain foods, and the attention you received, or did not receive, as a result of these symptoms.

Psychotherapy can help you to examine the connection between your own emotions, and unresolved conflicts, and how they may be affecting your food allergies. Even if a direct cause-and-effect relationship does not exist, your emotions may still make you more susceptible to food allergies. With a psychotherapist, you can explore the experiences you had as a child, and situations you are facing now as an adult, and begin to see connections, if they exist, with your food allergy. You can learn to better cope with fear and anger, and avoid, for example, an upset stomach or irritated colon that may be further exacerbated by eating the foods that set you off.

Psychotherapy can be a long-term process. While you may experience some psychological relief after a few sessions simply because you are spending time with a caring and helpful person, understanding yourself better and learning more effective coping methods takes time. Try to find a therapist who has worked with individuals with eating disorders, or with individuals whose emotions often lead to physical symptoms. And make sure this is an individual you trust and with whom you feel comfortable.

Reflexology

As with other branches of Chinese medicine, reflexology treats food allergy by clearing the digestive system of a buildup of toxins that has resulted in blocked energy, leaving the major digestive organs out of balance with the rest of the body. Because of these imbalances, the digestive system is oversensitive, with certain foods being reacted to as allergens, causing gastrointestinal upset, rashes, and other symptoms. While heredity and other factors may also be related to food allergy, reflexology attempts to reestablish the flow of energy along the meridians of the body, and detoxify and rejuvenate the organs, as well as provide relaxation. As a result, symptoms may occur less often, and be less severe. Reflexology is described in more detail in Chapter 3.

If you visit a reflexologist for help with your food allergies the treatment will focus on bringing all the organs and systems of your body into balance. The reflexologist will massage all of your reflex points, not only the ones that correspond with organs involved in digestion. The reflex areas that are most sensitive indicate the organs that are out of balance, and these areas will receive extra attention. You will also be encouraged to eat a balanced diet, and rid your life of as much stress as possible, as a diet heavy in preservatives, and excess tension, also contribute to digestive problems.

The examples that follow illustrate how a reflexologist might treat your stomach and intestines. You may also want to try these techniques on your own, or with a partner.

The Stomach   Reflexology techniques focused on the stomach help it to work more efficiently by keeping the mucous lining healthy. In turn, the stomach is less likely to go into a reactive mode as different foods are introduced. Additionally, if the stomach is working smoothly, recovery from an allergic reaction will be quicker and more complete.

The reflex points for the stomach are located on both hands and feet, though because the stomach is located off-center, toward the right side of the body, the stomach reflex areas are larger on the left hand and left foot. The stomach reflex area on the left hand is located on the palm, right under the pads below the ring finger, middle finger, and index finger. It is a smaller area on the right palm, just below the index finger. The stomach reflex area on the left foot is on the sole, almost halfway down, between the toes and the heel. It extends from the big toe to the fourth toe. It is in the same position on the right foot, but is located only under the big toe.

When working the stomach reflex area on the left hand, use your thumb to massage the whole area in a circular motion. Start under the ring finger and move toward the index finger, pressing lightly the first time, and then pressing slightly harder each time, for a total of seven repetitions. Repeat the same motions on the right hand, but only under the index finger.

When massaging the left foot, use the same circular massage technique as you used on the left hand, starting under the big toe and moving outward toward the fourth toe. Repeat this outward massage movement seven times, slightly increasing the pressure each time. Also perform this massage on your right foot, but only in the area under your big toe.

When you try these exercises, don't forget to regulate your breathing. Inhale as you press with your thumb, and exhale as you release the pressure.

The Intestines   When the intestines are healthy, they are able to play their role in processing the food and ridding the body of waste matter. When the intestines are out of balance with the rest of the body, toxins can build up and stagnate. Food allergy symptoms can be more severe. Using reflexology techniques for the intestines can help heal them from the diarrhea and upset that often results from food allergy, and help detoxify them from the buildup of food additives that may be contributing to the food allergy symptoms.

The intestinal reflex areas on the hands start in the center of the palm and occupy the lower third of it in an area the shape of a square. In the feet, the intestinal reflex area is located on the sole, beginning at the top of the heel and extending up to just below the center of the foot, also in an area approximately the shape of a square.

To massage the intestinal reflex area in the hands, use your index, middle, and ring fingers and press firmly, using a circular motion, from the center of this area and working outward. Repeat this action seven times, each time increasing the pressure a bit more.

To massage the feet, use your thumb on the intestinal reflex area, using the same rolling motion as used on your hands. Begin in the center of the reflex area, and gradually work outward until you have massaged the whole area. Repeat this massage seven times. As before, begin with a soft touch, and then gradually press more firmly.

Massage the intestinal reflex area gently, on both your hands and feet. If you feel some tenderness, or pain, in this area, it is a sign that you have some distress in your intestinal track. This may be related to your food allergy. Continue massaging your intestinal reflex areas to release the blockages that are causing this distress.

Working with Reflexology Reflexology won't cure you of food allergies, but it can be helpful in revitalizing organs that have been depleted of energy as a result of your symptoms. For example, diarrhea or cramps can leave your intestinal tract out of sync with the rest of your body, and reflexology can help bring this area back into balance. If your food allergy results in skin-related symptoms like rashes or in nasal congestion, you may also want to review the reflexology sections in Chapters 4 and 9 to find out how to apply reflexology in treating these symptoms.

Reflexology is a gradual process. While you may feel relaxed after the first session with a practitioner, give the process time to regain the energy that years of food additives and other toxins have taken away.

Reflexology and Addiction

Addictive behavior is a way of rewarding yourself, with actions that cause you to hurt yourself. Addictive behavior also relieves stress, at least for a while. Reflexology also does both of these things. It is a self-affirming way of making yourself feel good without doing damage to your body and mind. And it is a great way to reduce stress, calming your mind and steadying your nerves so that you can cope with your daily life.

Regardless of whether your addiction involves food or alcohol, a regular visit to a reflexologist once or twice a week can provide a break to focus on meeting your own needs and returning to your own center, without the distractions of daily life. One of the health-giving aspects of reflexology is that it involves two people, with the practitioner communicating a compassion and concern without words. This communication can enhance your own sense of self-esteem and it is out of love for ourselves that we break addictive behavior patterns.

In addition to the use of reflexology in helping you to feel relaxed and centered, it can also be useful in treating the specific organs of your body that are affected by your addiction. You may even have caused yourself some physical damage from your addiction. Treating the pancreas with reflexology helps to keep the blood sugar regulated, which in turn lessens the desire for sugar and alcohol. Treating the liver and intestines activates the process of eliminating the buildup of toxins in the system, effectively cleaning your system out. Your moods can be more balanced through massaging the reflex areas associated with the adrenals. Treating the thyroid balances the metabolism.

Your reflexology practitioner will discuss your addiction with you and will begin an initial course of action to enhance relaxation and restore balance. It's a good idea to commit yourself to a regular routine of reflexology sessions, to help you stay emotionally centered. Remember that addictive behavior develops over a period of years, and overcoming it is also an ongoing process. You may want to learn a reflexology routine that you can practice with a friend, perhaps massaging each other. This can deepen your relationship and help you both to maintain a commitment to good health.

Shiatsu

Food allergy symptoms can be a reaction to an imbalance, such as an excess of toxins, in any organ of the body. Thus, your symptoms are unique to you. A qualified shiatsu practitioner will make a decision as to the exact nature of your food allergies and where they begin. Shiatsu treatment will then be focused on correcting these imbalances, with your practitioner using techniques aimed at correcting your condition and restoring energy and balance to your whole body.

Shiatsu massage can also be applied in treating the symptoms of food allergy, including diarrhea and abdominal pain. Because these symptoms can have a tendency to dehydrate the body, as well as prevent the assimilation of nutrients, the body can become debilitated. To prevent this debilitation, shiatsu treatment is aimed at stimulating digestion and regulating the operation of the intestines. As a result, any foods or toxins in the digestive system to which the body is reacting pass through more quickly. Shiatsu treatment for food allergy symptoms is focused both on the lower back, where the autonomic nervous system is controlled, as well as the shoulder blades, where the small intestine meridian is located.

The following are examples of how shiatsu is used in

treating food allergy symptoms. You may want to try these techniques with a partner.

Relieving Diarrhea and Abdominal Pain   A shiatsu technique for relieving diarrhea and abdominal pain begins with the receiver lying on his or her stomach. The giver first gently massages the back of the neck, just below the skull, then moves on to the points at the top of the shoulders, along each side of the spine, and on the base of the spine. From there, thumb pressure is applied to each side of the buttocks, to points along the side of the leg, to the ankle joint, and to a point at the base of the big toe of each foot. This is all done gently, though more pressure is applied on the leg and ankle points. After this, the receiver turns over and gentle hand pressure is applied to his or her abdominal area.

The result of this exercise should be at least moderate relief from the discomfort associated with diarrhea and abdominal distress.

Stimulating Digestion and Relieving Anxiety   The shoulder blades are crossed by the small intestine meridian, which is associated with digestion. For this treatment, the receiver lies on his or her stomach.

First, massage the ridge of muscles along the top of the shoulders. This area often carries excessive tension. The best way to massage this area is with the thumbs, one shoulder blade at a time, while you are sitting down and facing the top of the receiver's head. Place one hand on the shoulder blade and lay the thumb of the other hand along the top of one shoulder. Lean forward and press outward from the neck to the notch in the shoulder joint.

From here, work lower down on the shoulder blades. Place one hand on the receiver's shoulder, and with the other hand lean one elbow into the groove on the other side of the spine. Work down the whole area between the shoulder blades, then change hands to work on the other side of the spine.

Also try placing foot pressure on the shoulders. Sit back away from the receiver's head, and support yourself with your hands behind you. Place your feet on top of the receiver's shoulders, and tread lightly.

These treatments can, as discussed previously, be useful in relieving specific symptoms. However, for ongoing relief from food allergies, it is best to schedule a consultation with a shiatsu practitioner who can determine where the imbalances are in your body that may be resulting in food allergies. After these imbalances are determined, you will meet with the practitioner for regularly scheduled sessions in which shiatsu techniques will be applied to promote healing.

Before undergoing shiatsu, have a talk with your physician. While you may be sure about the causes of your food allergies, it is important that your physician support this method of treatment. It may be a good idea to get a checkup first, especially if you have been experiencing any new symptoms, to make sure that you don't have any new ailments. For example, shiatsu is not recommended if you have appendicitis, peritonitis, pancreatitis, ulcers, a twisted bowel, contagious diseases, or an intestinal obstruction. Once your physician agrees that you are up to it, then visit a practitioner and give it a try.

Shiatsu practitioners may also make diet recommendations to help you avoid symptoms, including cutting back on meat and dairy products, and eating more whole grains, fruits, and vegetables. Shiatsu is also compatible with acupuncture and herbal medicine.

Twelve-Step Groups

Twelve-step groups have their roots in Alcoholics Anonymous, which is organized around the twelve steps that are required to attain sobriety, beginning with the admission of an uncontrollable addiction. Proponents of Alcoholics Anonymous believe that alcoholism is the result of an allergy to alcohol—a physiological condition—that can only be treated through avoidance. This concept has recently been adopted for use in treating other problems, including obesity, troubled relationships, and addiction to other drugs.

Twelve-step groups are helpful in a number of ways. They aid you in gaining insights into your addiction, including what situations cause you to become self-destructive and what alternate behaviors you have at your disposal. They provide you with a support group of others who understand your problems because they are experiencing similar concerns. Twelve-step groups also help you to understand your spiritual side as you define your higher power and learn to rely on this power as you face life.

If you feel your food allergy—and you can include alcoholism as an allergy—is causing you to behave in a self-destructive manner, you may want to check out an Alcoholics Anonymous or an Overeaters Anonymous group. They are free of charge, and are scheduled often, even nightly, in most regions of the country. Simply look for the name of the organization in your local telephone book, and call for a schedule, or contact your community mental health office.

Visualization

One of the best ways to treat your food allergy symptoms is with relaxation, and visualization can be useful in aiding your relaxation by keeping you focused on healing images. Begin your visualization by consciously relaxing, telling each part of your body, from head to toe, that it is time for it to relax. Inhale and exhale in a calm, easy rhythm. Meditation techniques can help with this.

When you begin to feel relaxed, begin introducing pictures to your consciousness.

Create an image of your gastrointestinal system. Imagine your intestines looping around and around, pink and vibrant, calm and stress free. Imagine any toxins in your system being pushed along the intestines, until they are gradually released from your system. Imagine yourself free of pain and distress.

When visualizing for food allergy symptoms, focus on any images of peace and calm that work for you. Imagine healing colors. Or wild animals gradually becoming quiet and docile. Think of quiet beach scenes, or imagine yourself sitting in a clearing in the middle of the forest.

Learn to relax, then begin imagining situations from your past in which you felt secure and happy. Once you teach yourself to relax and create positive visualizations, you can begin targeting your visualizations toward new situations you want to create in your life.

Yoga

Yoga, which is described in Chapter 6, is an excellent means of relaxing your entire body. Hatha yoga, one of the more popular forms of yoga, stresses the importance of body and mind awareness, and teaches various breathing and relaxation techniques to achieve this awareness. Hatha yoga techniques include deep, lung-expanding breathing. The effects of yoga are both immediate and cumulative: a few minutes of yoga positions and breathing can provide you with immediate relaxation, as well as a sense of well-being that can carry you through the day.

Glossary

Adrenaline A hormone released by the adrenal glands during times of stress. Also referred to as epinephrine.

Allergen Any substance that causes an allergic reaction.

Allergenic Used to describe any substance that causes an allergic reaction.

Allergic reaction A response to an allergen.

Allergy An immune system response resulting in oversensitivity to specific substances to which an individual has been exposed. An allergy results in symptoms such as sneezing, wheezing, skin rashes or eruptions, and swelling, diarrhea, and many other common and less common ailments.

Allergy shot The injection given as part of desensitization treatment for allergy. The injection includes a small amount of specific allergens to which the individual being treated is allergic, with the goal of "wearing out" the allergy over time.

Anaphylactic shock A severe allergic reaction, involving the entire body, with symptoms that include extreme breathing difficulty. Anaphylaxis can result in death.

Antibodies Proteins produced by the immune system in response to foreign proteins, including allergens.

Antigen A foreign substance that can cause an allergic reaction but is harmful to only some individuals.

Antihistamine A drug that stops allergic reactions by counteracting the effects of histamine.

Asthma The condition that results when the bronchial tubes are obstructed due to enlarged mucous membranes, producing symptoms that include coughing, wheezing, and shortness of breath.

Contact dermatitis   A skin rash that results from touching certain allergens.

Dander   Microscopic scales from the fur or feathers or skin of an animal, which can cause allergic reactions in humans.

Eczema   An itchy, dry, scaly skin rash caused by allergies.

Hay fever   A seasonal (spring and summer) allergic reaction, generally caused by pollen, with symptoms such as sneezing and itchy, runny eyes and nose.

Histamine   A chemical contained in certain cells of the body that, when overproduced due to allergy, causes the symptoms of an allergic reaction. Symptoms caused by histamines include runny nose, bronchial constriction, and skin blotches or welts.

Hives   Itchy red welts accompanying an allergic reaction. Also referred to as urticaria.

Inhalant   Microscopic airborne particles that, when breathed, can result in allergic reaction.

Mite   A microscopic insect that lives on human and animal skin and feathers, and collects in places like mattresses, upholstery, and carpets. Mites are also a component of house dust.

Mold   A fungus that produces microscopic spores that, when inhaled, can result in allergic reaction.

Pollen   The microscopic spores from grasses, flowers and trees that, when inhaled, can result in allergic reaction.

Pollutant   Airborne substances that irritate the respiratory tract.

Rhinitis   Inflammation of the membrane lining the nose.

Stress   Any internal or external factor that overly strains the bodily functions.

Urticaria   Hives, or red welts on the skin, resulting from an allergy.

Natural Medicine Resources

American Academy of Allergy and Immunology
414 East Wells Street
Milwaukee, WI 53202
(414) 272-6071
(800) 822-ASMA

American Academy of Environmental Medicine
P.O. Box 16106
Denver, CO 80216
(303) 622-9755

American Association of Acupuncture
    and Oriental Medicine
4101 Lake Boone Trail
Suite 201
Raleigh, NC 27607-6528
(919) 965-7546

American Association of Certified Allergists
401 East Prospect Avenue
Suite 210
Mount Prospect, IL 60056
(312) 255-1024

American Association of Naturopathic Physicians
P.O. Box 2579
Kirkland, WA 98083-2579
(206) 827-6035

American Association of Orthomolecular Medicine
900 North Federal Highway
Suite 330
Boca Raton, FL 33432
(407) 276-6167

American Chiropractic Association
17 Clarendon Boulevard
Arlington, VA 22209
(703) 276-8800

American Dietetic Association
216 West Jackson Blvd.
Chicago, IL 60606-6995
(800) 877-1600

American Foundation for Alternative Health Care,
    Research and Development
25 Landfield Avenue
Monticello, NY 12701
(914) 794-8181

American Holistic Medical Association
2727 Fairview Avenue East
Suite B
Seattle, WA 98102
(206) 322-6842

American Lung Association
1740 Broadway
New York, NY 10019
(212) 245-8000
(Or call your local chapter listed in the telephone book)

American Massage Therapy Association
National Information Office
1130 West North Shore Avenue
Chicago, IL 60626
(312) 761-2682

Asthma and Allergy Foundation of America
1125 15th Street, N.W.
Suite 502
Washington, D.C. 20005
(202) 466-7643
(800) 7ASTHMA

Center for Medical Consumers
237 Thompson Street
New York, NY 10012
(212) 674-7105

Human Nutrition Center
6303 Ivy Lane
Greenbelt, MD 20770
(301) 344-2340

International Academy of Nutrition
    and Preventive Medicine
P.O. Box 5832
Lincoln, NE 68505
(402) 467-2716

International Institute of Reflexology
P.O. Box 12462
St. Petersburg, FL 33733
(813) 343-4811

Integral Yoga Institute
227 West 13th Street
New York, NY 10011
(212) 929-0586

National Accreditation Commission for Schools and Colleges
    of Acupuncture and Oriental Medicine
8403 Colesville Road
Suite 370
Silver Spring, MD 20919
(301) 608-9680

National Asthma Education
  Program Information Center
4733 Bethesda Avenue
Suite 530
Bethesda, MD 20814-4820
(301) 951-3260

National Center for Homeopathy
801 North Fairfax
Suite 306
Alexandria, VA 22314
(703) 548-7790

National Commission for the Certification of Acupuncturists
1424 16 Street NW, Suite 501
Washington, DC 20036
(202) 232-1404

National Institute of Allergy and Infectious Diseases
9000 Rockville Pike
Bethesda, MD 20205
(301) 496-2263

Herb Sources

Annandale Apothecary
7023 Little River Turnpike
Annandale, VA 22003

Boerick and Tafel, Inc.
1011 Arch Street
Philadelphia, PA 19107
or
2381 Circadian Way
Santa Rosa, CA 95407

Boiron-Borneman, Inc.
6 Campus Blvd.
Bldg. A
Newton Square, PA 19073

John A. Borneman and Sons
1208 Amosland Road
Norwood, PA 19074

Ehrhart and Karl
17 North Wabash Avenue
Chicago, IL 60602

Herbarium
264 Exchange Street
Chicopee, MA

Horton and Converse
621 West Pico Blvd.
Los Angeles, CA 90015

Humphreys Pharmacal Company
63 Meadow Road
Rutherford, NJ 07070

Keihl Pharmacy, Inc.
109 Third Avenue
New York, NY 10003

Luyties Pharmacal Company
4200 Laclede Avenue
St. Louis, MO 63108

Mylans Homeopathic Pharmacy
222 O'Farrell Street
San Francisco, CA 94102

Running Fox Farm (flower essences)
74 Thrashing Hill Road
Worthington, MA 01098
(413) 238-4291

Santa Monica Drug
1513 Fourth Street
Santa Monica, CA 90401

Standard Homeopathic Company
204–210 West 131 Street
Los Angeles, CA 90061

Washington Homeopathic Pharmacy
4914 Delray Avenue
Bethesda, MD 20814

Weleda, Inc.
841 South Main Street
Spring Valley, NY 10977

Acupressure Points

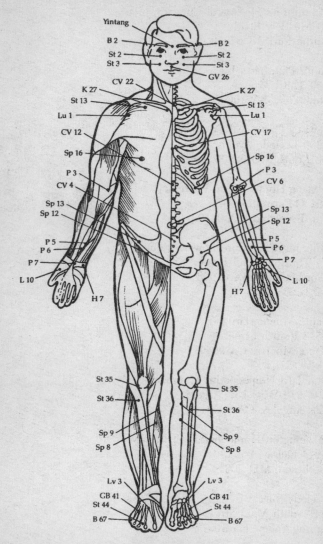

Front View

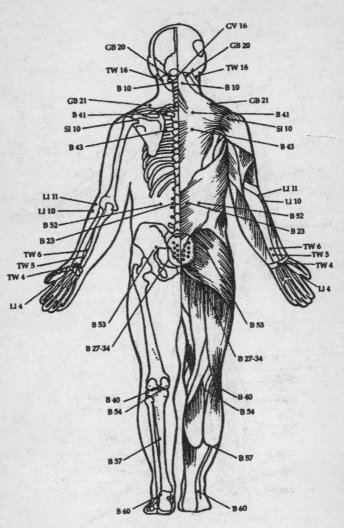

Back View

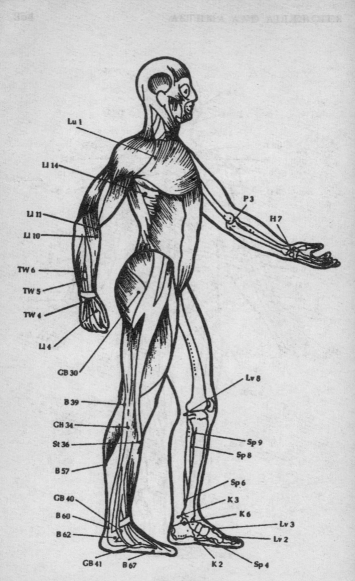

Lu 1
LI 14
LI 11
LI 10
TW 6
TW 5
TW 4
LI 4
GB 30
B 39
GB 34
St 36
B 57
GB 40
B 60
B 62
GB 41
B 67
K 2
K 3
K 6
Sp 6
Sp 8
Sp 9
Lv 8
P 3
H 7
Lv 3
Lv 2
Sp 4

Side View

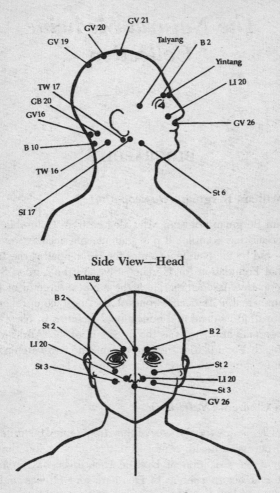

Side View—Head

Front View—Head

The Natural Medicine Collective

BIOGRAPHIES

Dr. William Bergman *(Homeopathy)*

William Bergman holds an M.D. degree from Columbia University and has completed postgraduate physicians' programs sponsored by the National Center for Homeopathy, the International Foundation for Homeopathy, and the United States Homeopathic Association. He is the medical director of Hahnemann Health Associates, one of the most comprehensive homeopathic medical and educational facilities in New York. Dr. Bergman also serves as the president of the World Medical Health Foundation, Inc., an organization researching the cause, treatment, and prevention of disease.

Brian Clement *(Nutrition)*

Brian Clement is the director of the Hippocrates Institute, the first progressive health center in this country. A founding director of the Coalition of Holistic Health, he has served as director at health centers in Denmark and Greece and has consulted at holistic clinics throughout the world. With over twenty years of international leadership experience in the field of alternative health care, he has appeared on numerous radio and television shows and has conducted hundreds of workshops and seminars on natural medicine.

Dr. Brian Fradet *(Chiropractic, Panel Coordinator)*

Brian Fradet holds a doctorate of chiropractic from the prestigious New York Chiropractic College and has completed postgraduate research in neurology at the New York University Medical Center. He is a longstanding member of the American Chiropractic Association, the Foundation for Chiropractic Education and Research, the Parker Chiropractic Research Foundation, the New York State Chiropractic Association, and the Chiropractic Federated Society of New York. He is the founder of the Fradet Pain Clinic in New York.

Elaine Retholtz, L.Ac. *(Acupuncture)*

Elaine Retholtz is a licensed acupuncturist and a diplomate of the National Commission for the Certification of Acupuncturists. She is a graduate of the Tri-State Institute of Traditional Chinese Acupuncture. She holds a master's degree in nutritional sciences from the University of Wisconsin-Madison. She maintains a private practice in New York specializing in acupuncture. She is the supervising acupuncturist for Crossroads: An Alternative for Women Offenders—A Project of the Center for Community Alternatives (formerly National Center on Institutions and Alternatives/Northeast).

Dr. James Lawrence Thomas *(Psychology)*

James Lawrence Thomas is a licensed psychologist and neuropsychologist with postdoctoral certificates in cognitive, relationship, group, and brief therapy. He is on the faculty of the New York University Medical Center and has served as the consulting neuropsychologist to Mt. Sinai Medical Center's Department of Neurology. He holds degrees from Yale, the University of California, Berkeley, and City University of

New York. Dr. Thomas maintains a private practice in New York.

Dr. Maurice H. Werness, Jr. *(Naturopathy)*

Maurice H. Werness, Jr., received a doctoral degree from the Bastyr College of Naturopathic Medicine. He is the medical director of Healingheart Healthcare, one of the West Coast's most prominent facilities for holistic care. He is also the director of development at the Institute for Naturopathic Medicine. A former tennis professional, Dr. Werness is the founder and director of True Tennis, an organization that teaches tennis and health education to physically and emotionally challenged people.

Gary McLain, Ph.D., is a freelance writer specializing in contemporary issues. He lives in New York City.

Index

Acupressure, 3, 27–29, 123–
    124, 141–144, 181–182,
    215–217, 251, 281–282,
    313–314, 348–349, 384–
    387
Acupuncture, 3, 10, 23–27,
    79–85, 141, 217–218,
    314, 349
Addiction, 355–358, 370–371
Affirmations, 124, 144–145,
    182–183, 218, 251–252,
    283–284, 314–315, 350
Allergens, 70–73
Allergic rhinitis and hay
    fever, 74–75, 128–173,
    179, 190–191, 199, 201–
    202
Allergy shots, 154, 163, 179,
    203
Anaphylactic shock, 4, 181
Angelica, 146, 224, 238, 351
Animal allergy, 135–136
Anise, 291–292, 353
Antibiotics, 198, 200–201,
    264
Antibodies, 69–72
Antihistamines, 153, 164,
    179, 181, 203
Apis, 193, 324–325
Aromatherapy, 3, 85–89,
    145–147, 183–185, 219–
    221, 252–254, 284–287,
    315–318, 350–352
Arsenicum album, 155, 191,

    193, 196, 231, 260–261,
    295, 296, 325, 361
Aspartame, 342
Asthma, 208–245
Astralagus, 149

Baths, 34–38, 317, 318
Beck, Aaron, 51
Behavioral therapy, 50–51
Belladonna, 196, 294, 361
Bergamot, 316–317
BHA/BHT, 342
Biofeedback, 9, 10, 53–55
Black pepper, 224
Botanical medicine, 3, 10,
    38–43, 89–106, 147–
    151, 185–189, 221–226,
    254–257, 287–293, 319–
    322, 352–359
Breathing exercises, 226–
    228, 257–258
Burdock, 290, 320–321, 327,
    357

Calamine lotion, 192, 323
Carbohydrates, 57–58
Cayenne, 292–293, 353
Cedar, 147, 220, 285
Chamomile, 260, 286, 317,
    327, 351, 354
Chi, 21–25, 28–29, 79, 82,
    121, 127, 168–169
Chiropractic, 10, 43–44
Cognitive therapy, 51

Colocynthis, 196, 361

Coltsfoot, 224–225

Comfrey, 188, 321

Contact dermatitis, 74, 192–
193, 296–297, 308–309,
323, 324

Cortisone, 200–201

Couples therapy, 51

Croton tiglium, 192, 296–
297, 324

Currie, James, 34

Cypress, 220, 385

Damiana, 149

Decongestants, 153, 179,
181

Detoxification, 113–114, 163

Dust allergy, 135, 138–139

Eczema, 74, 178, 183, 188,
193, 200–201, 311, 313–
314, 326, 327

Elimination diet, 116–118,
165, 177, 178, 199–200,
202, 204–205, 239, 326,
328, 363, 365

Emotions, 78, 83–84, 137,
180, 213–214, 249–250,
310–312, 339–340

Endorphins, 24–25

Enemas, 104, 112

Enkephalins, 24–25

Environmental pollutants,
68–69, 77, 110–112,
137, 214, 249, 273–307

Ephedra, 163, 201–202,
237–238, 265

Eucalyptus, 220–221, 224,
254, 257, 285, 289

Euphrasia, 155–156, 191

Exercise, 28–29, 64–67,
124–125, 228–229, 258–
259, 301

Family therapy, 52

Fasting, 112–114

Fats, 57

Fiber, 58

Fitzgerald, William, 46

Five-element theory, 22

Food additives, 61, 115, 137,
162, 177, 205–206, 236,
239, 264, 266–267, 342–
344

Food allergies, 73–74, 115–
118, 162, 177–178, 193–
196, 198–200, 202–203,
248–249, 310, 335–375

Freud, Sigmund, 49

Galvanic skin resistance
(GSR), 53

Gate theory of pain, 25

Gestalt therapy, 50

Ginger, 187–188, 189, 223–
224, 235, 256, 288–289,
354–355

Ginko, 149–150, 225

Ginseng, 302

Hahnemann, Samuel, 15–16,
29, 30, 106

Hay fever (see Allergic
rhinitis and hay fever)

Headaches, 282, 294–295

Herbal medicine (see
Botanical medicine)

Herb sources, 382–383

Heredity, 73, 76–77, 136–
137, 140, 174, 313, 339

Hering, Constantine, 32, 106

Hering's Law of Cure, 32–
33

Hippocrates, 14–16, 34

Histamine, 71, 72, 211, 300,
310, 339

Hives, 74, 178, 193, 309–
310, 326–328

Homeopathy, 3, 9, 10, 15–17, 29–33, 106–110, 153–156, 189–198, 230–233, 259–264, 294–297, 322–325, 358–362
Hydrocortisone, 192, 323
Hydrotherapy, 17, 33–38
Hypnosis, 10
Hyssop, 253

Iatrogenic illness, 13, 40
Immortelle, 147, 286, 317
Immune system, 69–73, 97–98, 153, 175, 176, 298, 339–340
Immunoglobin E (IgE), 71, 211, 339
Inorganic allergies, 273–307
Insurance companies, 10, 44, 46, 53
Ipecac, 196, 232, 261, 296, 361

Jasmine, 317–318
Journal writing, 125, 234
Juvenile allergies, 174–207
    allergic rhinitis and hay fever, 179, 190–191, 199, 201–202
    food, 177–178, 193–196, 198–200, 202–203, 248–249
    skin, 178, 185, 188, 191–193, 199–201
Juvenile asthma, 246–272

Kniepp, Sebastian, 35

Lavender, 254
Lemon, 220, 318
Leukotrienes, 71, 264, 265
Licorice, 321–322, 327
Liver, 297, 299–300
Lust, Benjamin, 17

Lymphocytes, 69

Macrobiotics, 10, 78, 125–126, 156–159, 235
Marshmallow, 290–291, 321
Massage, 3, 10, 34, 44–46, 125, 151–153, 229–230, 293
Mast cells, 71, 211
Meditation, 3, 4, 28–29, 126, 159–161, 235–236, 301, 303, 325, 362
Meridians, 23, 27, 44, 121
Minerals, 58–59, 300
Mint oil, 352
Modeling technique, 51
Molds, 133–134
Monosodium glutamate (MSG), 239, 343
Moxabustion, 24
Mustard seed, 150

Naturopathy, 15, 17, 110–114, 162–164, 198–204, 236–238, 264–266, 297–303, 325–328, 362–364
Neurotransmitters, 86–87
Nitrates/nitrites, 343
Nutrition, 9, 55–63, 78, 114–120, 164–165, 204–206, 238–240, 266–267, 328–329, 364–365
Nux vomica, 295

Operant conditioning, 51
Oriental medicine, 9, 20–29
Orthomolecular medicine, 63–64

Pain, 24–25
Palmer, David Daniel, 43
Parabens, 343

Peppermint, 150, 354
Perls, Fritz, 50
Pesticides, 68
Petrochemicals, 277, 278, 280
Physical medicine, 9, 43–47
Pollens, 128–133
Preissnitz, Vincent, 34–35
Preservatives, 68, 115, 162
Prostaglandins, 71, 214
Protein, 56–57
Psychiatry, 52
Psychoanalysis, 49–50, 52
Psychotherapy, 9, 47–53, 126, 165–166, 207, 267–269, 329, 365–366
Pulsatilla, 231–232, 261, 295
Purging, 102

Recommended Dietary Allowances (RDAs), 63
Reflexology, 3, 46–47, 120–123, 167–168, 240–241, 269–271, 303–306, 330–332, 366–371
Relaxation, 10, 53, 54, 301, 328
Resources, 19, 378–381
Rhus toxicodendron, 192, 323–324
Rosemary, 221, 286

Sabadilla, 155, 190, 193
Scheel, Joseph, 17
Self-help groups, 10
Serotonin, 86–87
Shiatsu, 44–45, 126–127, 168–171, 241–242, 371–373
Skin allergies, 74, 178, 185, 188, 191–193, 199–201, 308–334

Skullcap, 163, 202, 238, 266, 355, 356
Spiritual healing, 10
Spirituality, 78
Spongia, 232, 261–262
Stimulating herbs, 97–99
Stress, 78, 214, 249–250, 299–302
Succussion, 31
Sulfites, 215, 267, 343
Sulfur dioxide, 236, 239, 264
Susceptibility, levels of, 11–12
Swedish massage, 44, 45

Tai chi chuan, 28–29
"Taking the case," 13–14, 107–108
Thymus gland, 298
Tonics, 100
Tranquilizing herbs, 99
Twelve-step groups, 374

Urtica urens, 193, 324

Vegetarian diet, 236–237, 264–265
Visualization, 3, 78, 127, 172–173, 242–244, 271–272, 301, 306–307, 332–334, 374–375
Vitamins, 56, 58–59, 237, 264, 265, 300, 364

Wyethia, 155, 190–191, 193, 295, 325

Yin and yang, 21, 81, 157, 217
Yoga, 127, 161, 244–245, 307, 375

Zang-fu, 21–23